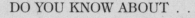

DO YOU KNOW ABOUT . . .

- The most popular newspaper for the hearing-impaired?
- The best movies to see and truly enjoy?
- The easy manual alphabet that hearing friends and family can use to help a hearing-impaired "dropout" return to the hearing world?
- The biggest "don't" for a hearing spouse?
- How to select the most helpful telephone?
- The simple instructions to give service and delivery people *before* they arrive?
- The home furnishings that provide the best environment for the hearing-impaired?
- Common medications that may damage hearing?
- New possibilities for reversing hearing impairment?

DISCOVER ALL THIS AND MUCH MORE IN

WHEN THE HEARING GETS HARD

"This book will save thousands of 'ears'!"
—Robert B. Brummett, Ph.D., Professor of
Otolaryngology and Pharmacology,
Oregon Hearing Research Center, Oregon Health
Sciences University,
Portland, Oregon

When the Hearing Gets Hard

Winning the Battle Against Hearing Impairment

Elaine Suss

Foreword by
Ruth R. Green
Executive Director Emerita
League for the Hard of Hearing

Bantam Books
New York • Toronto • London • Sydney • Auckland

WHEN THE HEARING GETS HARD

PUBLISHING HISTORY
Insight Books hardcover edition / 1993
Bantam mass market edition / September 1996

ISBN 0-553-57469-8

Published simultaneously in the United States and Canada

Bantam Books are published by Bantam Books, a division of
Bantam Doubleday Dell Publishing Group, Inc. Its trademark,
consisting of the words "Bantam Books" and the portrayal of a
rooster, is Registered in U.S. Patent and Trademark Office and in
other countries. Marca Registrada. Bantam Books, 1540
Broadway, New York, New York 10036.

PRINTED IN THE UNITED STATES OF AMERICA

OPM   10 9 8 7 6 5 4 3 2 1

With enduring love to

Virginia Louise, Adam Benjamin, Rebecca Elizabeth,
Anna Rose, and Andrew Samuel, who manage
language thoughtfully because
they want their grandmother
to understand all their words

Contents

Introduction

BY JOSEPH WERSHBA

Elaine Suss, a masterful researcher, has researched the dickens out of her own condition of hearing impairment so that anyone who has ever suffered from this disorder, anyone who has a parent, a mate, a child, or a friend with this disability can know the bottom line: (1) What are the forms of hearing impairment? (2) What can we do about it for ourselves or for others around us who have to deal with hearing impairment?

In my years as producer for CBS television's *60 Minutes* the stories that affected me deeply were about people who had been devastated by humiliation—and fought back: the young athlete who could no longer move her arms and legs because she had been paralyzed in a car crash but who fought back to "walk" again, with the aid of muscle and nerve stimulation; the people who were called lazy, dumb, or stupid because they couldn't read—until it was discovered that the light that hit the page or hit their eyes was preventing them from reading the letters, a condition that could be corrected with the aid of properly colored lenses; the 55-year-old salesman who fought back when he was discharged with the excuse that he was no longer "up to snuff" but really was discharged before he could reach the age where his pension would be guaranteed.

Elaine Suss is this kind of fighter. This is a remarkable book by a remarkable woman. I wish I had had this book 30 years ago. My mother suffered from a growing and severe loss of hearing. She didn't know it and neither did the family until late in the game. I should have had an inkling when she complained about Harry Reasoner, one of my colleagues on *60 Minutes*. "Harry talks between his teeth," my mother said. "He never moves his lips. I don't understand what he's saying."

Sure, Harry Reasoner kept a stiff upper and lower lip, but his speech pattern was clear and easily understood by all, I thought. My mother was sending out the distress signal of every person who is hard of hearing; she was watching Harry intently on television in order to read his lips. She did this instinctively, not even realizing she was compensating for not being able to hear adequately.

After you read Elaine Suss, you will never again talk to a hearing-impaired person through lips that don't move distinctly.

My mother was getting mixed signals. The loneliness that so often accompanies hearing impairment was causing her to turn more and more to the "magic box" for company, but she couldn't get the messages straight. In her loneliness and despair she lashed out against, of all people, Seiji Ozawa. "Why does that Japanese fellow keep playing the same Tchaikovsky piece all night?" She was referring to Ozawa and his Boston symphony. "Doesn't he think I had a cultural upbringing and that I know more than the *March Slav* he and his orchestra keep playing over and over again!"

We finally took my mother to Dr. Sam Rosen, whom you will meet in this book. Dr. Sam, a giant in his field, told my mother sympathetically, "I'm afraid your hearing nerves are just about gone."

"But why?" my mother asked him in consternation, unwilling to believe.

"Because, my dear, at our age the nerves tend to wear out."

"At your age," my mother shot back. "Not mine!" My mother was sixty-five. Dr. Rosen was seventy.

My mother was fitted with hearing aids, which helped some, although she found putting them into her ears a torturous process.

Later, when she had a heavy chest cold, my mother was taken to a local hospital. A doctor and nurse decided to keep her in the hospital overnight. Not understanding their words, fearful and panicky, my mother became obstreperous. She insisted on going home. The doctor prescribed a common but potent tranquilizer to calm her nerves. The dosage was too potent. My mother was never the same again mentally. She died within the year. How much better she would have fared had she not been afflicted with severe hearing loss and had she heard the doctor and nurse and not needed a tranquilizer to calm her we will never know.

I read my mother's story on every page of this book. I read my own insensitivities on every page. Most of all, I read hope on every page.

So pay strict attention to Elaine Suss's spade work on this question of drugs: Be wary of drugs that may be ototoxic, drugs that under ordinary circumstances are benign but when taken by a person with hearing impairment may produce disastrous results.

The problem is there, widespread, and under conditions of noise and debilitating sounds, the problem grows. Elaine Suss does not shrink from describing the pain. Even her husband, with sensitivity and deference to her difficulties, takes a beating now and then. It is an honest, unsparing book. But Elaine Suss comes as a healer. Every month brings new technology to help the afflicted hear more than they heard the month before. Listed are devices that may help you, what they cost, and where you can buy them.

Equally significant is the healing that is yours without price: understanding, patience, thoughtfulness. Care that is useful. Attention that is not patronizing. If you suffer from hearing impairment, says Elaine Suss, you have hard choices to make. But you can do it. Acknowledge your own impairment; don't wait for others to do it for you. Make clear rules about how you will communicate with others when you have passengers in your car. Educate your callers on the telephone about your special needs for keeping conversations simple. Learn how to deal with your grocer and your hairdresser—and, for God's sake, don't let her start cutting your hair until the two of you are agreed on exactly how far you want her to go!

More from Elaine Suss: Express gratitude to those who show thoughtfulness. If your spouse is hearing impaired, learn how to talk directly and simply and, again, don't patronize. And—in what may be a new finding from Elaine Suss's research—if one of your ears is completely dead, use hearing aids for both ears anyway. For some reason it works better. And again, urge your doctor to prescribe drugs very carefully and to keep a check on the results.

You'll find chapter after chapter in this book detailing almost every possible aspect of hearing impairment, information for those afflicted, for those who deal with the afflicted, and for the doctors who work with them. You'll find repetition here. Naturally. If you don't repeat, how will you learn? Elaine Suss is a teacher. She is a poet and creative writer, and so she tells the story with lyrical clarity. And when humor applies, she applies it.

Elaine Suss has given a gift to all of us in *When the Hearing Gets Hard*. The book is a Magna Carta for the hearing-impaired and for those of us who are not but who will always have to deal with it.

Foreword

There are over 28 million people in the United States with some degree of impaired hearing. While it is one of the more prevalent disabilities, it continues to be the one that is least understood by the general public. Hearing impairment is a hidden disability, and all too many people, themselves hearing impaired, prefer to keep it that way. Hearing impairment is the only disability that puts a major responsibility on the non-disabled person; it becomes the hearing person's responsibility to be sure that the person with impaired hearing understands the communication. Receiving the message can vary, depending on the degree of hearing impairment, the ability of the person with impaired hearing, and the compensatory aids the person with impaired hearing employs. All too often, the person with impaired hearing rationalizes the situation with, "If only they would speak more clearly." Yes, there is a responsibility to try to speak clearly; however, the process is a two-way street, with responsibilities for both the hearing and the hearing-impaired partners.

A hearing loss can't be corrected with a quick fix; a person with a hearing loss requires a program of rehabilitation—hearing aids, assistive devices, speechreading, listening training, and assertiveness training (i.e., how to take responsibility to access communication). During my

12 years as executive director of the League for the Hard of Hearing, I've met many of the 15,000 people with impaired hearing the league provides services to annually. I've also had occasion to talk with their families and am keenly aware that the person with normal hearing needs to learn appropriate communication strategies to be sure he or she is understood by the person with impaired hearing. And so I welcome this book by Elaine Suss.

Only in a partnership, with each assuming appropriate responsibility, can we have effective communication between the 28 million people with hearing impairment and people with normal hearing. Based on her own experiences, Elaine Suss provides strategies to promote this communication partnership.

RUTH R. GREEN
EXECUTIVE DIRECTOR EMERITA,
LEAGUE FOR THE
HARD OF HEARING

Preface

When people determine that they have a hearing loss, their response is often to pretend the problem doesn't exist or to assume that nothing will help them. And yet, hearing loss affects every aspect of our lives—social, emotional, family, and work. Some psychologists say that losing one's hearing is the single most traumatic event that an individual can experience.

As a hard-of-hearing person who lost my hearing gradually during my late twenties and thirties, I experienced firsthand the emotional and practical adjustments that someone with hearing loss must make to remain a viable member of the hearing world. At the time my hearing began to change, I had family responsibilities, a demanding job, and a network of friends—but I knew very little about hearing loss. When I began searching for tools to help me, a book like this one—written by someone who had personally experienced the complexities of hearing loss—was not in print.

Through a series of lucky events, I stumbled upon Self Help for Hard of Hearing People (SHHH), the national organization of and for people of all ages and all levels of hearing loss. SHHH is dedicated to providing hard-of-hearing people and their families with the information that they need to successfully address the personal challenges of hearing loss. Our members understand that there are productive steps they can take to improve communication and, importantly, that there are millions of people who have experienced the challenges they must meet every day.

Elaine has written this book from the same perspective that we at SHHH have always tried to present. She gives us technical solutions and describes situations in which those solutions have been helpful to her and others. She shows us that hearing loss is not a simplistic problem that is easily resolved. It is this aspect of her book that is perhaps most valuable.

Too often people have been led to believe that there is a quick fix for hearing loss. Elaine shows us some workable solutions that have helped her. She provides an enormously useful compendium of information (technological, medical, social, psychological, legal, family-related) that will encourage readers—both hard-of-hearing people and their families—to productively address their hearing loss and then move on with their lives. We are proud that one of our memebers has developed a book to affirm a philosophy that has provided hope for SHHH members and will provide inspiration for many more people.

DONNA L. SORKIN
EXECUTIVE DIRECTOR
SELF HELP FOR HARD OF HEARING PEOPLE, INC.
7910 WOODMONT AVENUE
BETHESDA, MD 20814

Author's Introduction

Separated from the hearing world by ear disorders, we are often lonely. Unable to handle our difficulties, some of us become self-pitying and "drop out." There are ways to minimize our isolation, ways to manage the consuming challenge, ways to bridge the widening gap between our world and the world of the hearing.

This book offers some of the many paths we can take to happy reunion with our hearing friends and family and suggests ways we can find new companionship with others who share our disability. The book is also a guide for the friends and family of people with hearing disabilities, a guide to help them understand a world very different from their own.

And this book is also a guide to the prevention of hearing loss. It documents cases of hearing impairment that could have been avoided. It says to the hearing community, "Be careful, there are shelves filled with medications that can destroy your precious organ of hearing. Study the lists prepared with assistance from our country's outstanding scientists and physicians in the field. Those of us in the world of hearing impairment do not want your company here." And it says to people with already impaired hearing, "Study the lists of medications in this book that can further damage your hearing. Question your doctors about prescriptions and their potential for hearing harm. There are often alternative medications that are safe."

Most everyone has had some contact with a hearing-impaired person. Nevertheless, for families and friends of people with hearing impairment, this affliction remains mystifying. Unlike blindness and other visible disabilities, hearing impairment is a bully, daring the hearing to put a best foot forward to help, demanding that the hearing change their normal behavior patterns, insisting that the hearing school themselves in nuances that take great effort.

When members of the seeing world confront the blind, instinct makes them alert to what needs to be done: helping them navigate through traffic, leading them safely past or around physical obstacles. Ever mindful of the blind one's incapacities and limitations, a seeing person who is sitting with a blind friend before a bowl of red and golden delicious apples would not tell the blind person to choose a golden apple. Nor would the seeing person suggest to the blind person that they watch television or ask the blind person's opinion of a friend's new hair arrangement.

And who in the world of the unimpaired would ask a paraplegic to join a game of football or tennis? The blind and the legless need not explain their limitations once, let alone over and over again, as the hearing impaired are compelled to do.

Even the hearing mate of a person with hearing impairment needs constant reminders about how to interact. My husband is a thoughtful, considerate, and loving man, yet he often forgets how to deal with my hearing impairment, which has been severe for many years. I must constantly remind him about my difficulty in understanding a normal flow of language, a normal interchange of ideas, simple questions and answers. Even as I write this book—and he helps in a thousand ways, for example, with telephone queries, an essential ingredient of my writing—he blunders in dealing with my impairment. He returns from walking our dog Yogi and tells me he met our new neighbor and her little girl. "How old is the child?" I ask. "Well," he answers, "old enough to ask about the kind of dog Yogi is." He says this as he laces his shoe, so I see very few words. I understand the word *about* and conclude that the child is about a certain age. When I lift his face to see his answer repeated, I need to remind him that he should answer my questions directly. A simple, direct answer, not a philosophical or humorous or sarcastic or judgmental one, is what people with severe hearing impairment require.

This brief interchange is just one small example of how hearing impairment imposes new or altered behavior on the friends and family of people with hearing disabilities. In this book I offer many of my own experiences and those of other people who are hearing impaired in the hope that the hearing world may better understand our invisible affliction and become better able to deal with it.

And in this book I offer my hearing-impaired comrades the many lessons I have learned in order to "make it" in the hearing world, especially the need for patience and understanding of the hearing who really want to befriend us but aren't always sure of the best methods and approaches. People with hearing impairment must teach the hearing lovingly and gently about our special needs.

Acknowledgments

Many people helped shape this book and, in the hardcover publication of 1993, I acknowledged these friends. Now I express thanks to friends who helped immeasurably as I updated *When the Hearing Gets Hard* for paperback.

My friend/husband, my ear to the hearing world. Ruth R. Green, Executive Director Emerita of the League for the Hard of Hearing, encouraged me even before chapter one of *When the Hearing Gets Hard* was written. Her suggestions for the *When the Hearing Gets Hard* paperback updating have been invaluable. Donna Sorkin, Executive Director of Self Help for Hard of Hearing People (SHHH), was always available to discuss the updating of this book with me; she has been most giving of her time and excellent advice. Hundreds of members of SHHH have written, thanking me for putting their many feelings into words, and they have been generous with information about medicines they suspect to be causes of their hearing difficulties—information that was of tremendous help for my update of deafening medications. Steve Malawer, Audiologist and Hearing Aid Dispensary Manager at the Hearing and Speech Center of the Long Island Jewish Medical Center, was instrumental in providing the most current information about assistive aids. Dr. Robert Brummett and Dr. Leo Parmer were unsparing of their time in helping to update chapters 11 and 12; these chapters represent the most current medical data about medications that can cause hearing disorders.

Chapter 1

Conflict and Confusion

When Hearing First Gets Hard

It is my own hearing impairment that has made me aware of the strain hearing impairment can put on the friends and family of the impaired. My own impairment has also made me understand the impaired who do little to help themselves out of their lonely detachment from the hearing community. I want to share with them some of my own experiences and those of other hearing-impaired people and describe for them the many ways hearing impairment can be managed. I also want to detail the many ways the hearing community can help.

The wedge hearing impairment can drive between two communities of otherwise congenial people makes me think of impairment as a villain appearing either suddenly and violently or stealthily, like a lengthening shadow.

The villain can be intimidating to both the hearing and the impaired. But it can be contained, permitting the two communities to interact and nourish each other. I have seen this happen. I have also seen the despair when it does not happen.

The National Institute on Deafness and Other Communication Disorders (1989, April) reports that 28 million Americans are affected by hearing impairment, so there is scarcely a family or a hearing person untouched by the problems of hearing disorders. And no one is immune to this affliction. It can happen to anyone—young, old, rich, poor. In recent years it has been happening in larger numbers to both young and old.

After ten years of progressive impairment, I became one of the 7.2 million Americans (Hotchkiss, 1989) with significant bilateral loss, a condition that gave me great difficulty understanding what was being said in normal conversation even when I wore two hearing aids.

This severe loss, which shut me out of the hearing world in which I used to enjoy full participation, made me feel like half a person. I tried selling myself on the bromide that it is better to have had and lost than never to have had at all. I would enumerate for myself the wonders I'd enjoyed in preimpairment days, the operas, lectures, movies, poetry readings, concerts, adult education courses, conversations with friends and family in restaurants—on the telephone, at social functions, while walking on an avenue, while driving in a car or other conveyance—and remember the convenience and pleasure of listening to cassettes at museums, listening to the radio, and watching whichever TV program I was interested in. Instead of feeling better because I once had what now I'd lost, I felt confirmation that I was reduced to half a person.

Knowing there was nothing that could really replace that lost half of me, I'd dream of the day of a miraculous transplant—maybe the donor auditory organ of a human or even the organ of a dog.

Finding myself unable to enjoy full participation in the hearing world was painful, but most painful of all was the experience of being excluded from the hearing world by friends. I'm sure the hearing are unaware of the sensitivities of the newly hearing-impaired.

"She won't be able to hear," a once good friend told

another as they discussed getting tickets to a Broadway play. I read their words and felt myself choking with sadness at being excluded from a theater party in so cavalier a manner. I spoke up—too sharply, I think: "That's a decision for me to make." Outraged, I stomped away.

True, my loss has severely cut into the pleasures of the theater, but it has not made the theater absolutely off-limits. I have found ways, though complicated, of continuing this pleasure. At any rate, it is not for others to decide what my loss prevents me from doing.

During the initial period of bereavement for my loss, I investigated mechanical devices to help me regain some of that other half of my person. I also adjusted preimpairment routines. And I found new ways of relating to family and friends in the hearing world.

Regaining what I can of that lost half of me is a constant challenge, but it can be done. I've seen many others, impaired as severely as I, do it too.

How Recognition Happens

The room filled with voices is often the place awareness first happens. It is where it happened for me. Standing amid a hum of voices, recognizing few of the words pouring from fast-moving lips, I felt as though I were watching a film being projected from a failing machine. Several happenings like this and I knew the film projection was fine. The failing machine was my ears.

At first I tried to dismiss this failing. When the hearing-impaired person doesn't acknowledge early signs of the problem, the problem is often caught by a family member or close friend. In my case it was my son.

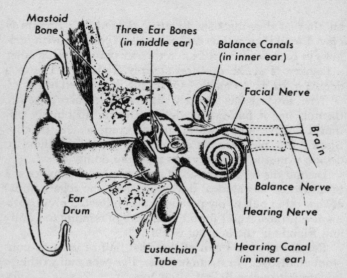

FIGURE 1. The ear is divided into three parts: the external ear, the middle ear, and the inner ear. (Courtesy House Ear Clinic, Inc.)

Family Friction

"What's the matter, Mom?" My son spoke with deep concern. It was our family Thanksgiving dinner, and I kept asking people to repeat themselves.

"It's the dining room," I told my son. "Something about this large table."

"What do you think, Dad?" he asked.

"Well, I've been suggesting for a while now that she see about her hearing."

"Listen," I said, waving the drumstick I'd been enjoying, "this is a celebration. First time in six months we're all together. And it's Thanksgiving. We have so much to be thankful for." I looked around the table at my daughter and son-in-law, who had flown in from Michigan for the holiday, at my daughter-in-law, who was nursing our first grandchild, at my sister and her new husband, who had driven three and a half hours to be with us.

My husband said, "It would be more of a celebration and we'd all be thankful if you did something about your problem. Remember the other night at the concert? You didn't even hear them make the announcement about the program change."

I felt my cheeks ablaze. "That's absolutely unnecessary, and I'd appreciate it if we could just enjoy the dinner I worked on for two days."

"Okay," my husband agreed, "but please stop shouting."

"I'm not shouting," I insisted. At the same time, I worried that perhaps I *was* talking louder than necessary, though it didn't seem to me that I was.

My sister and brother-in-law were clearly embarrassed. My son got up to come to my side of the table. Putting his arms affectionately on my shoulders, he said, "I'm sorry, Mom. It was dumb of me to start this. I just don't want my mother to be holding a big horn in her ear."

"We all get old," I said.

"Not you," my son answered with his typical humor and a big smile. "You're only thirty-nine and a bit."

"Thanks dear, now let's just drop it." The fact that a beautiful dinner was getting no attention because my ears had become the star attraction made me flush with annoyance.

My daughter said, "A hearing disorder is nothing to be ashamed of, Mom. You know you could get some help."

"I will. I promise. I'll make an appointment. There's a new hearing aid store on Main Street."

"Mom, I mean you should get some counseling. People can get help, and then they're better able to handle their infirmities."

I was ready to laugh and cry at the same time. My daughter, not yet finished with her master's degree in counseling, was already practicing her future profession on me. I had to leave the table to digest the fact that my family had seized this festive occasion to let me know what must have been on their minds for some time. It had certainly been on my mind, although I had closeted the knowledge in some far corner of myself, hoping the problem would go away. It didn't, of course. In fact, it was becoming distressingly more apparent.

In sadness and anger I retreated to the kitchen. This should not have been a day for problem solving. When I returned to the dining room with my special pumpkin pie, I said, "Well, we had my ears for the entree. Now who wants whipped cream on the pie and who wants to be noble?" That did it. Everyone laughed good-naturedly, and we finished dinner as a happy family—everyone except me because, for the first time, I saw myself living in a world apart from the people I loved most. Even the nursing baby, my darling granddaughter, would sing out her first words to all ears but mine.

Havoc at the Hairdresser

Nothing makes me appear very different from the other women who crowd into Cut & Curl this February morning. Nothing at all, until it is my turn to take one of the seven chairs in front of the head-washing basins, step one in the hour-long procedure that organizes my hair for the week. Once I greet Sally, the woman who will shampoo and towel-dry me in preparation for the snipper and blow-dry person, I am set apart from the women occupying the three seats to my left and the three seats to my right: I am the only one who does not participate in friendly chatter with either Sally or the women on either side of me. Unless I have explicit instructions for Sally, like "Please rinse a little more; I still feel soapy," I am deadly quiet.

This is not because I am an introvert or snob. I remain quiet because I have removed my hearing aids, and with my head tilted back into the washbasin I cannot see Sally's or the other women's lips. When two-way conversation is impossible, people with hearing impairment remain mute.

Once I am seated in Alice's chair, in the snipping and blow-dry section, I socialize a little. Hearing aids remain in my handbag since blow-dryers as well as water ruin these expensive instruments, but I can see many words in the wide mirror I face. If Alice would not pirouette or chat face-to-face with other hairdressers, I could make out most of her words.

Alice's habit of turning her head and pirouetting while working on my hair causes disaster this particular February morning. Dancing gracefully behind me, she says, "Why don't we do a nifty boyish-fifties? Be gorgeous on you."

Seeing some words, guessing at others, I think she says, "It's heading up for the fifties. Gorgeous February we're having." "Yes," I say enthusiastically. "Just what the doctor ordered. I'm catching a noon flight to Chicago for an interview."

Alice's scissors fly. A whirlwind wounding the countryside. A tornado. I am a tree. Truncated. Uprooted. There is no saving the left side of me. "Put down those scissors!" I shriek. "Don't cut another hair!"

Actually, the boyish-fifties does look nifty. But I refuse to have the right side of my head shorn. There will be nothing to conceal either hearing aid. It's not that I am vain or embarrassed. I make no secret of my hearing disability. But I like to make the announcement in my own way. I never want my husband to tell people, "My wife can't hear you. She's hearing impaired." Neither do I want the bulbous pink plastic filling my ears to make the announcement for me.

When my hearing first became a problem, my husband

would tell people who spoke in a whisper or indistinctly, "My wife doesn't hear well, so please talk very slowly and clearly." He meant to be helpful, but each time he took over this way I would feel incompetent, mentally deficient. Sometimes I would see a pitying look in the eyes of the person my husband was advising. Sometimes a hurt or embarrassed look, as though they had committed an indiscretion. After my husband's announcement many people would address the conversation only to him. Some, trying to include me, would shout. Shouting can be worse than whispering for people with hearing impairment.

I decided it was best to make my own announcement. I say to people I am meeting for the first time, "I have a hearing problem." When they make the comment, "Oh, I'm sorry," I quickly answer, "I do well if you look directly at me and talk slowly." Explaining my impairment myself puts people at ease, makes them a partner in my difficulty. They work at talking slowly and clearly. They often become interested in how my impairment happened. Some confess they too have a slight problem and ask about my aids and my audiologist. Some complain to me about relatives who cannot handle their disability and ask for advice. Making my own announcement is reassuring to new acquaintances. They are pleased that they can converse with me. We become equals. The gap between our worlds closes. I do not want my husband or hearing aids to announce my impairment.

This morning at Cut & Curl is unfortunate. Alice does her best to reconcile the boyish-fifties on the left side of me with the girly lengthy-twisties on my right side. I leave the shop tentatively, hoping and praying that the hearing-impaired, body-building actor I am going to interview in Chicago will be too absorbed watching my mouth to notice the strange thing that has happened to the top of me.

In a Taxi

The taxi ride to the airport is time for quiet reflection. When I must communicate with the cab driver, my questions are carefully worded to elicit a one-word answer.

The moment I enter the taxi, even before I give instructions about my destination, I explain my hearing impairment and show the driver how to raise a hand and one finger to indicate yes and how to turn his thumb down if the answer is no. The thoughtful driver will move his head along with his finger. Asking a cab driver to reply "Correct" or "Negative" is expecting too much of this person weaving through traffic. Even if the driver should remember to say "correct" or "negative," cascading vehicular noise would blur those otherwise useful words.

The two-way radio is jarring, each blast a reaffirmation that I am a prisoner of my disability. I sit stiffly and hope the roaring, which sounds like angry jungle beasts, is not some emergency that will direct the cab driver to detour and make me late for my plane.

I remove a mirror from my handbag to inspect Alice's innocent damage to half my head. It is easy for people with hearing impairment to succumb to paranoia. It takes great effort on my part to erase the thought that Alice should be faulted for being so quick to snip away at me. The fault, I know, was mine. I know too that from such misunderstandings many a good laugh will follow.

Flying

I explain my hearing impairment when I make flight reservations. Airlines are eager to help the hearing disabled and encourage the impaired person to give all pertinent information about connecting flights and services that may be required upon landing. They are prepared to assist with telephoning to hotels, contacting taxi companies, and making other necessary arrangements. Airlines advise people with hearing impairment where to report when arriving at the airport. A hostess guides the hearing-impaired person to the flight gate and then places the person in the competent and willing hands of a flight attendant.

When I travel I take full advantage of the Americans with Disabilities Act—legislation that gives people with hearing impairment access to facilities and services available to hearing people. The day I make a hotel reservation, I request a phone with volume control, a television set with closed captioning, an alarm that is placed beneath my mattress to shake me awake, a fire and smoke alarm with flashing lights.

Preparing for a flight, I follow my otolaryngologist's advice and use the nasal spray Beconase AQ for two weeks prior to my flight. Beconase AQ is a cortisone-type spray and, to be effective, should be used twice a day for the two weeks. The day of my flight I take a Dristan tablet, the aspirin-free decongestant.

These medications, plus swallowing and other procedures followed once the plane begins its descent, are attempts to keep the eustachian tubes open. Other methods of keeping these tubes open include yawning and the Valsalva maneuver, which involves pinching the nostrils closed while keeping the mouth shut and attempting to blow breath through the closed nostrils. The Valsalva maneuver can open the eustachian tubes; however, excess pressure is inadvisable. The maneuver should be learned from a doctor. The medications too should only be taken when recommended by a doctor.

Ears need special protection from the pressure changes that occur from the time the plane reduces altitude until it lands. Again, it is the helpful flight attendant who checks with the pilot and informs me when the plane is to begin its descent. I arm myself with apples to be chewed, small bites at a time, in order to keep swallowing. Some may prefer chewing gum or sucking hard candies. I find that chewing an apple is more pleasant for this period of time, which can vary from 20 minutes to the better part of an hour, depending on the length and other conditions of the flight.

My travel handbag is as well equipped for my ears as it is for the interview I am about to do. In addition to decongestants and apples, I carry spare batteries for my hearing aids, a rain scarf and umbrella to protect my hearing aids in the event of rain, and a portable phone amplifier, which is always with me. It must be every hearing-impaired person's nightmare to be unable to use a phone in an emergency. Excellent portable telephone amplifiers are available at Radio Shack stores. For better listening under difficult conditions, I also keep my Williams Personal FM System (described on pp. 91–92 and illustrated on p. 93) in my travel bag.*

The plane glides smoothly this beautiful February day. In this economy-class section, I get first-class treatment, which is particularly appreciated when announcements are made. Words through the loudspeaker are siren alerts to my damaged ears, worrying me that the plane is in trouble. The thoughtful flight attendant appears at my seat regularly with explanations about weather reports and estimated landing time.

---

* The audiologist at the Hearing and Speech Center at the Long Island Jewish (LIJ) Medical Center explained how to enjoy movies on long flights. "To plug into the movie on an airline, some commercial earphones may work. Earphones distributed by the airlines don't carry sound loud enough without distorting. The highest quality earphones are the Sony Professionals, which are larger. I've used them for many years. They are the earphones used by recording engineers and can be both loud and clear. They cost about $90. They are available at Sam Ash and at audio stores used by professional musicians."

Adjusting my food tray when lunch snacks are wheeled toward my seat, I am aware that the stewardess is staring at my new hairdo. "Do you like it?" I ask.

"It's nice," she says politely. "What is it called?"

"Half and half. I guess."

She smiles and goes on with her duties. I open my notebook to review questions I will ask Lou Ferrigno this afternoon. He is a young people's idol, a hero to aspiring bodybuilders. He has been severely hearing impaired since he was three years old, yet he became Mr. Teenage America, Mr. America, Mr. Universe, and Mr. International. He starred in *Pumping Iron* and became "the Hulk" in *The Incredible Hulk.* He had a speaking part in *King of the Beach* and was Hercules in *Hercules* and the *Adventures of Hercules* and Johnny Six in the TV series *Trauma Center.* I will interview him in a sports equipment store, where he will be promoting his bodybuilding program.

Havoc on the Job

I am in the midst of a crowd of fans waiting their turn to enter the store to see, maybe touch, the amazing body of Lou Ferrigno. There is anxious milling about. This young man they worship has run out of photographs to autograph. Suddenly, there is squealing and shoving. The beautiful body is emerging. I shove a little too, trying to introduce myself: "I'm Elaine Suss. I've looked forward to meeting you."

Lou Ferrigno nods pleasantly and continues walking. "We have an appointment to do an interview for my book about hearing impairment," I call up to him as he quickens his pace toward a limousine parked down the street. I overhear fans complaining that they got photocopied pictures because earlier fans went into the store twice and got two good photographs, so I reason that the Incredible Hulk is rushing to the limousine for additional photographs.

Running alongside those tree trunk legs, I call out, "It's almost four o'clock. Do you think our interview will be delayed?" I get a smile and a nod as Lou Ferrigno opens the shimmering silver limousine door and vanishes.

Like some of his young fans, I bang on the street-side darkened window. "We have an appointment," I say, my voice loud and worried. There is no response and the chauffeur has turned on the ignition. I rush to the front of the mammoth car. "Please," I implore the chauffeur, "I've come all the way from New York for this appointment. I do have an appointment with Mr. Ferrigno. Please." My body is flung over the silver hood. "Please, I've waited a month for this interview. It's for a book about hearing impairment."

The chauffeur communicates by phone with the rear of the car. The back door is opened slightly, and I am yanked inside by a beautiful woman—Lou Ferrigno's wife. "I thought you weren't showing," she says and sits me in the jump seat, knee-to-knee with the Incredible Hulk.

This is one of the problems people with hearing impairment have. I cannot always handle phone conversations myself. My husband sometimes stands next to the phone to listen for what I may not understand (and this is not a foolproof method). Setting up interviews with prominent people may involve 20 or more calls. Some calls are handled by my husband at his office when I am not present. Many people must clear the calendars of celebrities like Lou Ferrigno. Everyone is busy. Words are brief.

Lou Ferrigno does not use the telephone. He was told about the interview and expected it to take place inside the limousine. I expected it to take place inside the store.

When I approached him, he understood nothing I said; thinking me another fan, he merely nodded politely.

Driving to another part of the city, we do the interview. Someday I'll tell my grandchildren about it, and I'll tell them how their grandmother climbed atop a limousine to accomplish it.

Chapter 2

The Helpful Home

Keeping Impairment from
Getting the Upper Hand

The failing ear deserves the same consideration any other part of the body would get were it to fail. The eyes, for example, that can no longer read fine print. The back that aches. And, like other troubled parts of the body, the failing ear may need only minor adjustment or assistive aid or may be correctable with surgery or medication. The failing ear may also be a warning signal of neurological or other major problems.

The roomful of unheard or misheard voices is a tap on the shoulder suggesting that something be done. Consultation with an ear specialist—an otolaryngologist or otologist—is *step number one*. If it is determined that the problem is *sensorineural,* contacting an audiologist with good credentials is *step number two*. *Step number three* is learning to keep impairment from getting the upper hand.

Hearing impairment made me feel like a stranger to myself. I had to get reacquainted. I am a writer, spending most days at home, and my house was no longer working for me. Things I once took for granted—the doorbell, the telephone—became impossible to deal with. I had to learn

15

to make the impossible possible, to keep impairment from getting the upper hand.

Telephone Assistive Devices*

In 1989 New York Telephone workers left their jobs because of a dispute involving health benefits. Life without easy access to a telephone and its information services was so intolerable that the *New York Times* ran a front page story quoting people as saying, "It's just been hell." A hearing-impaired friend said to me, "It's always hell for people with hearing impairment. At least the telephone strike is temporary."

The telephone is one of the largest monsters I had to learn to live with. This piece of household equipment frequently requires more patience than reasoning with a willful child. It can consume more energy than washing windows and sweeping floors. It can also give people with hearing impairment, as well as their families and friends, the best laugh of the day.

Now fitted with various assistive devices, the telephones in my home accommodate my impairment. To maximize the benefit of these assistive devices, my hearing aids have T (telephone) switches. I keep a supply of hearing aid batteries on hand but it is very comforting to know that I can always purchase hearing aid batteries at one of the more than 7000 Radio Shack stores.

* For information (manufacturer's name, address, phone number; cost of item) on these and other aids, see the Directory of Resources at the back of the book. Keep in mind that the assistive equipment described in this book barely scratches the surface of what is available. To guide readers to what is out there waiting to help impaired ears, there are several excellent sources of information; see Publications for the Hearing-Impaired in the Directory of Resources.

The Amplification Wheel

The amplification wheel, capable of increasing volume by 30 percent, is contained in a small cutout on the underside of a special telephone handle, the Volume Control (VC) Handset, between the receiver and mouthpiece. The wheel is rotated to boost or lower volume.

Many, many hearing-impaired people are acquainted with the amplification wheel, but there are methods of using the VC Handset that can considerably improve the wheel's performance. Not all telephones enable the VC Handset to give satisfactory results. When my impairment required an amplification wheel, I searched for an old-model (and therefore heavy) rotary phone. The newer (lightweight) touch-tone phones were not as efficient. Finding an old-model telephone, into which a VC Handset can be plugged, is a task. Family or friends may have one for you, and in appreciation you can buy them a new lightweight model. You might even advertise in a local newspaper.

Using the VC handset is not the simple matter of putting receiver to ear. Different voices require different methods of using the VC Handset. Voices vary widely. Differences in pitch, emphasis, enunciation, evenness, speed, word separation, and breathiness fall differently on different ears. In addition to the quality of the voice, there is the temperament of the person behind the voice. Some people switch voice range when they are not quickly understood. Others will flatten their voices or overexaggerate in their eagerness to be understood.

For certain voices I need a hearing aid as a companion to my VC Handset; with others a hearing aid plus a VC Handset causes too much distortion. When a VC Handset is used, with or without a hearing aid, the unused ear should be made inactive. If the unused ear does not wear a hearing aid, it should be covered with a hand. If the

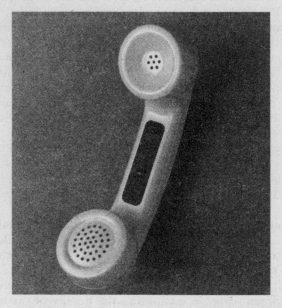

FIGURE 2. The AT&T handset with amplification wheel

unused ear wears a hearing aid, the aid should be shut off.

Studying voices and choosing the appropriate assistance is only part of the amplification procedure. The VC Handset with a hearing aid works differently when the receiver is held against different areas of the aid. Comprehension is most effective for me when I place the receiver of the VC Handset at the top of my aid, pressing the rim against my head with the receiver facing parallel to the floor.

The audiologist who supplies the hearing aid should be consulted about optimum placement of the handset. This placement depends upon the location of the microphone in the hearing aid. The location of the microphone may vary with the manufacturer, or with the style of hearing aid. In behind-the-ear hearing aids, the microphone is usually located at the top of the aid. In-the-ear hearing aids usually have microphones at the base. The user of an in-the-ear hearing aid would usually hold the handset in normal position but slightly away from the hearing aid.

When the VC Handset is used in conjunction with a hearing aid adjusted to its T (telephone) position, background noise is eliminated. Without an activated T switch, the hearing aid, which amplifies all sound equally, may be a necessary but troublesome companion for the VC Handset.

Ordinary household noises that are screened out by the normal ear—running water, a vacuum cleaner, the clicking together of dishes or silverware, the opening or closing of a door, footsteps—can cause tremendous telephone interference. The turning of a newspaper page, an incident not even considered noise to a healthy ear, can make it impossible for the hearing-impaired person to comprehend the voice at the other end of a phone. If a dog barks or a baby cries, the hearing-impaired person may have to excuse himself or herself from a telephone conversation. Even without noise interference inside the home, outdoor noise pollution from an airplane, an auto-mobile, or gardening equipment infringes on the quality of telephone reception for the impaired ear wearing a hearing aid that is not set on its T position. Adjusting my hearing aid to its T position is so effective that I can carry on a telephone conversation while standing between an operating dishwasher and my barking dog.

In addition to eliminating background noise, the T position protects against the whistle of a hearing aid that is set too high. With the T switch activated, I can set my aid at maximum with no concern that it will whistle. The T position also eliminates the metallic feedback that some-times occurs when the hearing aid touches the handset.

It is necessary to consider the person at the other end of the phone. If the hearing-impaired person uses the VC Handset together with a hearing aid and holds the VC Handset at the top of the aid in a position parallel to the floor for reception, as I must, it is important that the VC Handset be brought down to normal mouthpiece position for speaking. Radio Shack stores have a fine assortment of amplified sets (handsets with volume control). They also have phone extension bells and flashers that turn lights on and off when a phone rings.

The Portable Amplifier

The portable amplifier is a convenient alternative to the VC Handset. Battery-operated and weighing approxi-mately a quarter of a pound, the portable amplifier fits most conventional phones. Like the VC Handset, it boosts volume 30 percent.

I sometimes find it efficient to attach the portable am-plifier to a VC Handset. The amplifier is placed in direct contact with the listening-impaired ear just as a normal

ear would be positioned at a telephone receiver. It is then
adjusted to the volume needed to enhance the handset.

There is a minor inconvenience when using the portable amplifier for incoming calls: I have to ask the caller to
wait while I attach the portable amplifier to the telephone
receiver, and activate it. With the VC Handset, only the
simple activating of a T switch on the hearing aid is required. There is also the problem of having batteries
available and remembering to deactivate the portable amplifier when a phone call is completed. However, dollar-
wise, it is an excellent telephone assistive aid.

The Comtek Telephone Adapter

The Comtek Telephone Adapter is a very sophisticated
telephone assistive device. A special handset cord re-
places the original cord and plugs into a telephone
adapter that is attached to the base of the telephone with
a self-adhesive Velcro strip. I wear a neckloop transductor
plugged into a receiver companion that connects to the
adapter. When telephone switches on my hearing aids are
activated, I hear with both ears, through two hearing aids.
I no longer hear through the receiver.

Binaural hearing increases my comprehension on the
telephone tremendously. Voices that were not possible for
me to hear with other assistive devices are now heard.
With careful talkers who speak from acceptable telephones, I can usually have a decent conversation. For incoming calls there is the inconvenience of keeping the
caller waiting until I hook into my Comtek. But friends
and family are so appreciative of my competence with this
unit that they do not become impatient.

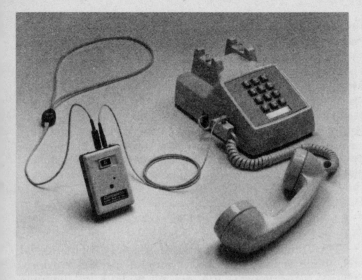

FIGURE 3. The Comtek Telephone Adapter

A Telephone Called Clarity

Just as vision loss is not always correctable with unselective magnification, so too is hearing loss not always correctable with unselective amplification. Clarity, a product of the Walker Equipment Plantronics Company, features a control panel that enables me to select the best volume for those frequencies that give me difficulty on other phones. Voices that become blurred when I raise the volume on other phones are intelligible on my Clarity phone. Clarity is a self-contained unit, but when more amplification is required, Clarity can be used with a hearing aid on its T (telephone) position. Clarity also has a lighted ringer with a flashing light alert.

Additional features of Clarity, which can be enjoyed by

the entire family, include a mute button that puts a caller on hold, a program for emergency and frequently used numbers, and a last number redial capability.

My home is probably a model of telephone technology for the hearing-impaired, but the instrument is still a monster, smothering me with words that make no sense and compelling me to keep phone calls so brief that I worry that I am losing the art of conversation.

When I initiate a call to a voice I am familiar with, I can choose the most suitable phone; other-initiated calls require guesswork. Incoming calls are most difficult. I grab the closest instrument and struggle to identify the caller. Dear friends struggle along with me, often spelling out their names letter by letter (e.g., "B as in boy"). I am grateful to these friends who don't hang up while I try to determine who they are, who patiently answer questions that may clue me in, who want to be understood just as I want to understand. People acquainted with my hearing impairment know that I must keep my phone calls simple and brief, that idle chatter is two-way frustration.

Not quite hearing or not understanding the voice at the other end of the wire makes me feel that I am drowning, desperately grasping for a world that is fading away, groping for straws to keep me afloat. There is, however, a sunny side to this telephone blight: the neighborhood telephone addict, who swamps my friends with nuisance and nonsense calls, has dropped me to the bottom of her list.

Even the best telephone assistive aid cannot work effectively if the voice at the other end mumbles, whispers, shouts, or speaks very fast or if the telephone is a low-powered fashion design. I can understand very little that comes through one of the original Princess phones and very little that comes from a cellular or cordless phone.

Family and friends at the other end of the line want to be understood and are eager to be accommodating, but we with hearing impairment must lead them gently. I make

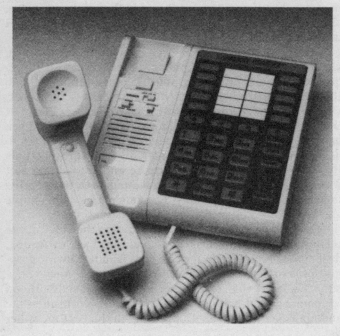

FIGURE 4. The Clarity telephone

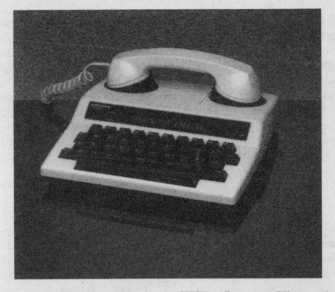

FIGURE 5. The Text Telephone (TTY) (Courtesy Ultratec.)

people aware of their pace and manner of speech by explaining that it is *my* ears that are at fault. Hearing people have sensitivities also. Because it may embarrass them to learn that their speaking habits can be improved upon, I quickly establish the fact that the fault is with my ears. Together we figure the pace of speech I require, how they can best talk for me to understand, which of their phones is most suited to my ears. They become partners with me in my troubled ear department, which can be great comfort for one who inhabits the lonely world of hearing impairment.

It is more difficult to make partners of strangers who call. All incoming calls are more difficult than outgoing calls for the person with hearing impairment. Understanding the name of the caller can be the hardest part of the telephone conversation. But if the person calling in is a family member or friend, there are usually ways I can get clues. I will ask, "Do you live in my neighborhood?" or "Have we met recently?" and other questions that can get a one-word answer. I ask the person to answer by saying "correct" or "negative," which are easier for me to understand than "yes" or "no." The incoming call from a service person, a business call, the unsolicited call—all can give extreme difficulty. I sometimes ask, "Do I know you?" I've asked this question of my husband and my children and very close friends. They understand.

The Speakerphone

The speakerphone, a common piece of office equipment giving binaural reception, can be a fine assistive aid for the person with hearing impairment. Hearing aids are used in normal fashion; there is no T-switch involvement.

The Answering Machine: My Best Telephone Friend

When it is absolutely impossible for me to understand who the caller is, I have a best friend who helps. I say to the caller, "I have very impaired ears. Please hang up and call again. Let the phone ring four times, and when my machine answers leave a message. I will get back to you." Then I telephone my husband's office and play the message back for him. My husband then translates for me. So really it is my husband plus the answering machine who are my best telephone friends.

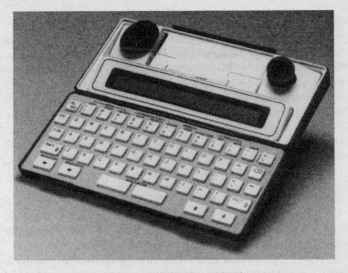

FIGURE 6. TTY by AT&T

The TTY: Text Telephone

The TTY: Text Telephone (TTY is the designation preferred by the hearing impaired community and the deaf community).

For people with extreme telephone disability, TTY is an excellent, never-fail assistive aid. The TTY is a typewriter with a display screen above the keyboard that shows the message being sent and the message being received. Above the display screen are acoustic cups into which the handset of your telephone fits.

How does the hearing-impaired person with a TTY communicate with a hearing person who does not own one? The impaired person types 800-662-1220 for the relay center in New York (see Telecommunications Relay Services Directory for numbers in all parts of the United States, page 258 of the Directory of Resources) and then types the telephone number of the person he or she wishes to communicate with. When the communications assistant types back to the TTY that the person to be communicated with is available, the hearing-impaired person types a message for the hearing person and waits to see the answer on his or her TTY. The hearing-impaired person and the hearing person word their messages, which they give to the relay center by TTY or orally, as though they are in direct contact with each other. Messages are not interpreted by the communications assistant; they are conveyed from one person to the other verbatim.

When communicating by TTY, I prefer using my voice for outgoing messages. For this combination of outgoing voice and incoming type you alert the relay operator by typing "I want a VCO (voice carry over) call."

The TTY manual has some instructions, but, as with most new assistive aids, I needed a guinea pig. My good friend Esther spent many hours receiving my TTY calls and trying to return messages for me to read on my display screen. Peculiar things happened. At times Esther's words would be clear on my display screen, but at other times the screen would display numbers, dollar signs, plus and minus signs. Those were frustrating hours for me, for Esther, and for the relay operator. Finally, the relay operator asked if my handset was set firmly into the acoustic cups. "How can it be?" I answered. "My handset has a square receiver and mouthpiece and the acoustic cups are round."

Now I know that the old adage was meant for TTYs; once I overcame the slips between cups and lips, that is, the air space that causes all kinds of difficulty, my TTY worked well.

How does the hearing person without a TTY communicate with a hearing-impaired person who owns one? The hearing person telephones the relay center in New York at 800-421-1220 (see Telecommunications Relay Services

Directory for numbers in all parts of the United States, listed in the Directory of Resources) and gives the assistant at the relay center the TTY number of the impaired person. If the impaired person is available, the communications assistant puts the message on his or her TTY. The conversation then proceeds with the communications assistant acting as a verbatim conduit.

How do two people with TTYs communicate? The caller dials the other TTY owner's phone number. The moment the first ring sounds, the caller activates his or her TTY and puts the handset into the acoustic cups on the TTY. The message appears on the display screen. From then on, the conversation is a result of two sets of fingers typing back and forth. There is no relay operator, no third-party factor.

The TTY has a personality most of those in the hearing world are not acquainted with. There is a need for slow speech, so the relay operator can transmit the message, and a need for patient waiting, while the message is being typed by the relay operator. To compensate for the delays, there is the satisfaction that everything said by the hearing person will be understood (read) by the person with hearing impairment. However, in this fast-paced world, particularly in the business world, some do not welcome a TTY phone call.

I've had a few unfortunate experiences. There is need in the hearing world for more knowledge about relay service. When the person with hearing impairment types a message asking the relay operator for a VCO, the relay operator tells the hearing person, "I have a VCO call for you. You will hear the voice of the person calling."

One hearing person who heard this message thought it was a solicitation and slammed the receiver down.

Another hearing person who heard this message shouted to his wife, "It's that deaf thing (meaning the service). Hurry up, we're in a rush." This response was from a very nice man. I'm sure he had no idea that every

word that can be heard by the relay operator is typed back
to the caller.

Yet another hearing person I wanted to interview said
to the operator, "What does she want?" The relay operator explained to this woman that I would talk directly to
her and that she should give her response slowly enough
so the message back to me could be typed. The woman
answered, "Well, let her tell me quickly." When I explained why I wanted to interview her, she continued
talking to the relay operator: "Tell her Thursday at ten for
half an hour."

I tried using the VCO to determine whether it would be
alright for me to tape the interview and whether my camera person could take some pictures. The woman kept
talking all the while I was talking so the relay operator
couldn't understand what she was saying. The operator
typed on my screen, asking me to tell the woman not to
talk while I was talking and to speak slower when she was
answering me. I didn't think the woman would appreciate
hearing that she was talking much too rapidly so I said
nothing about the pace of her speech. I did explain, however, that I always use two tape recorders and that my
camera person would come along with me.

I then explained a little more about the subject of our
interview so she would be prepared for it. The relay operator typed back to me that she thought I was put on hold.
I waited for several minutes until the relay operator typed
back to me, "I'm sorry, we were disconnected. Shall I call
back?" Since this was a woman in a great hurry I decided
it best not to call back. I had set up an interview and
basically that was what I wanted to accomplish. That
Thursday was disaster. The woman hadn't heard details
of the planned interview. Neither had she heard that I
would bring a camera person. With impatience she'd
given me an appointment and disconnected me. Her
sharp words sent me reeling. "I hate strange camera people. How dare you intrude this way."

There was no interview, only disappointment and insult. Fortunately, there have been very few of these experiences.

With patient friends and family, the TTY brings back the friendly chats, the harmless gossip that is nourishing on a dull day. The art of conversation, something I thought I had lost the skill for, has returned. Once again I am like other people in that fortunate world of the hearing.

Despite the few unsatisfactory experiences with the text telephone, it is an instrument that gives tremendous independence to people with hearing impairment. No longer is it necessary to rely on a hearing person to make difficult phone calls, calls that involve medical problems, calls to airports and bus terminals, calls to service companies where fast-paced voices frequently make it impossible to use other assistive telephone devices, all the phone calls that are part of doing household business. No longer is it necessary to rely on an assistant or secretary in the workplace.

AT&T gives special telephone call discounts to hearing-impaired owners of TTYs (approximate cost, $200). For those who make many long distance calls, the machine soon pays for itself, and thereafter there is the gift of discounted bills. For information about discounted bills, contact the telephone company in your area.

A Final Word on Using the Phone

Fitting my home with telephone assistive aids makes me a more efficient housewife, writer, and owner of Yogi, a West Highland terrier who frequently requires me to make telephone calls to arrange for a pet-sitter, to schedule appointments for periodic checkups with the vet, and

to solicit seasonal advice from the vet about allergy pills
and sprays.

For one of my many telephone calls to Yogi's vet, I used
my handset with amplification wheel. There was no time
to attach my Comtek telephone adapter, which requires a
neckloop transductor, connection into the special receiver, and connection from the attached adapter. Nor
was there time to use my TTY, which requires patient
waiting for an available relay operator.

The reason for haste with this particular phone call
was that Yogi had ingested the skin of a chicken neck to
which a needle was attached. (I'd been making a pocket of
the skin, a pocket that was to be stuffed and then sewn
shut.) As I was preparing the stuffing, the neck, needle,
and thread fell to the floor. Quicker than a flash, Yogi
grabbed the neck. My shrieks brought my cleaning man,
Frank, running from the back of the house. Together we
chased Yogi. When he was captured, he was contentedly
licking his lips (chicken skin is one of his favorites).
Frank had advice: "Give him some olive oil."

"Again with the olive oil," I said while grabbing my
Rolodex for the vet's phone number.

"Olive oil is the best." Whenever Frank caught me using corn or canola oil or soybean margarine, he came on
strong about olive oil. As I dialed, Frank kept insisting,
"Olive oil will make it slip right through him," while pat-
ting Yogi's head and believing him to be a doomed dog if
chicken neck and needle weren't followed with a dose of
olive oil.

Not even waiting for the receptionist to complete her
usual greeting, I said, "My Westie ate a chicken neck and
needle." Since Frank was so persistent, I added, "Should
I give him some olive oil?" I was sure I heard the receptionist giggle, though it could have been static, as she told
me to take it easy. This only made me talk more rapidly as
I demanded that she get advice from the vet about olive
oil.

"Just a minute," said the receptionist, adding something unintelligible. I assumed she wanted to answer another call, but I felt a needle coursing through Yogi's system had top priority.

Raising my voice, I said, "Listen, he ate a neck with a needle and thread. Should I give him olive oil?" She mumbled something, which infuriated me because she knew I was hearing impaired. I screamed for her to get the vet and tell him about the chicken neck and ask about olive oil. All I could make of her answer was that I should wait and take it easy. I turned the receiver over to Frank, saying, "See why this fool is telling me to wait, when a needle is wandering inside Yogi." Frank listened—for too long, I thought. Impatiently, I interrupted, "What is she saying?"

With a grin, which enraged me as much as the receptionist's demand that I take it easy and wait, he told me, "You've got the Chase Manhattan Bank."

Lesson: People with hearing impairment must be especially cautious to dial correctly.

The Doorbell

Listening for the doorbell can be a chore for a hearing-impaired person, but there are ways to make the chore easier. When I became severely impaired, waiting for a service person became a burden. A second bell at the back of my house was insufficient. If I was not in the very room with the bell, I would miss the service call. Then I learned about the buzzer, which, though not musical, is more efficient than a bell. Unfortunately, for a person with severe impairment, two buzzers still do not cover an average-sized house. More than two are counterproductive: each will lose enough volume to make three buzzers no more effective than two.

So when service people are expected, I have a routine. First, I explain my impairment. Unable to work with the usual span of time they insist upon—six to eight hours—I ask them to telephone approximately one hour before they will be arriving. Some comply; others do not, so I telephone *them* during the day. I also stress that I will definitely be at home and ask them to ring my bell (buzzer) several times and, if they get no response, to walk around my house and knock on windows. If a service call is extremely urgent, I leave my typing frequently to look for an approaching service van. An annoyance, yes, but think of all the healthy exercise. Actually, most service people are cooperative. Some will even telephone my husband's office if I do not respond to their telephone alert. My husband always manages to reach me.

Home Furnishings That Make a Difference

Sound bounces off hard surfaces, increasing confusion for people with hearing impairment. For us the most favorable environment includes wall-to-wall carpeting, soft sculptures, curtains and drapery, and upholstered furniture. Large open spaces are more difficult for the hearing-impaired than small enclosures. Separate rooms with thick doors are best. A solid kitchen door helps keep the noise of appliances from other parts of the house or apartment. Well-insulated ceilings help also. Small, round tables give the hearing-impaired a better view of a speaker's face and lips than do elongated rectangles.

Why then do I have polyurethaned-wood or tile floors? Window treatments that are either nonfabric blinds or nonfabric shades? Rooms that flow into each other with solid doors only in essential places like bathroom and bedroom? A rectangular dining room table?

Simple: I did my furnishing long before my hearing became impaired. And there are inconveniences many of us with hearing impairment prefer to live with.

I have, however, accommodated my impairment by acquiring area rugs and a collection of wall-hung rugs. Except for family dinners, I limit the number of guests at my dining room table to eight, and I sit in the middle of the long side of the table, a position that gives me the best opportunity to see faces and lips. I leave the host ends of the table to my husband and a guest.

There are assistive aids that can ease group conversation in the home. These and other assistive aids, discussed in various chapters, are listed in the Directory of Resources at the back of the book.

In learning how to make my home accommodate my impaired ears, I found some pleasant surprises along the way. Although running water is not kind to my ears, a tubful of still water is a new friend. I discovered this quite by chance when I was soaking in the tub and my husband needed information. Realizing that I don't wear hearing aids when bathing, he was careful to stand where I could see his mouth. Words that are usually difficult, even when I see a mouth, came through with startling clarity. I asked him to say something else on another subject. Again, I understood most words.

All hearing-impaired ears are not the same so I am not suggesting that all those with hearing impairment rush to immerse themselves in a tub of water, but my husband and I will now frequently delay a topic we want to explore until I am in the tub. Time after time the method has worked. Perhaps it is that my ears function better when I am in that relaxed state. Or perhaps it is because the bathroom is a snug enclosure: the small window glass is well covered, thick mats are on the floor, and large towels hang on the walls. At any rate, hearing impairment has added a super dimension to the bathtub in my home.

Household Harmony and Hearing Impairment

Congenial living requires effort by the hearing-impaired and the hearing. "So how do a hearing-impaired wife and her hearing husband really get along?" a friend asked me.

"Not always well. Now tell me how you and your husband, both blessed with good hearing, get along," I answered.

"Not always well," my friend admitted and we had a good laugh. Of course, I understood her question and because I think the difficulties between hearing and hearing-impaired mates can be eased with mutual effort, I'll explain my recipes for a happier home.

Early on, my impairment made me resentful when my husband had long telephone conversations with our children or friends and I, standing close by aching to know what was being said, was ignored. Since his mouth was hidden by the telephone, I could get no clues about content and therefore could ask no pertinent questions later. And once he completed a call, he would not always be able to give me a total report of what was happening with our daughter in Michigan or our son in Pennsylvania. Sometimes he would omit the very items I would have considered the most important or the most entertaining. Days later, he would recall some details, making me wonder how many other important items I'd never know about. I'd stand close to the telephone during these conversations and move his jaw toward me so that I could at least see some of his responses, which I hoped would suggest the subject being discussed and enable me to query him later. If the conversation appeared to be very serious, my anger would peak and I'd make continuous attempts to position his jaw. This was annoying to him and he'd wave me away with his elbow. At times we were reduced to a shoving match, with me shoving his jaw and him shoving my hand away.

I told my husband, "I bet the telephone in a hearing-impaired home causes more divorces than infidelity." I had not yet learned about those miraculous assistive aids: the Comtek Telephone Adapter and Clarity.

In those early days, however, I never gave up my right to grab for the ringing telephone first, but too often a family member or friend (though not all—and to those I am eternally grateful) would lose patience and ask if my husband was at home. There I'd sit, feeling discarded, even unloved, staring at the partially visible side view of my husband's lips for a clue as to what was happening in that exclusionary hearing world. When my husband spoke, with concealed mouth, to our little granddaughter, my eyes would brim with tears of self-pity and I would stomp out of the room.

Learning to cope with the telephone hazard was a painful process. My husband really made an effort to look in my direction while talking into the receiver. And we discovered the pad of paper and pencil. How simple! The moment my husband got to the telephone, I'd bring paper and pencil so he could make notes while he listened.

Then came Comtek and Clarity, and I became quite proficient at conversations when people remembered to pace their speech. Of course, there are always the complicated conversations that make me the outsider. But even then my Comtek adapter is helpful. I can be plugged into a conversation, which I hear through my hearing aids, and my husband can hold the telephone receiver in a normal position. I may miss many fast-paced words at the other end of the wire, but I hear my husband's voice with amazing clarity. The Comtek adapter and my hearing aids work together so remarkably that I understand my husband's speech better than when we have a face-to-face conversation. Being able to understand my husband's part of a phone conversation makes me a participant in the hearing world.

There are behaviors between husband and wife that may need to be modified when one of them becomes hearing impaired. For example, calling to each other from different parts of the home becomes a no-no. I cannot fault my husband. He's learned this restriction well. The fault is usually mine. Too many times I catch myself calling out to another part of the house from which I will never hear the answer. I am quick to apologize for this old habit.

Shouting to a hearing-impaired person is counterproductive. My husband knows this, but it is not always easy for hearing mates to control their exasperation when they think the hearing-impaired one should understand what is being said. I've solved this problem by showing, not telling. In a very noisy restaurant, I used no voice, forcing my husband to speechread (the current expression preferred to lipread). Recognizing how difficult it can be to read many words has increased my husband's patience when I am unable to see something he is saying.

The home is a happier place when the hearing spouse understands the best way to get the attention of the hearing-impaired one. When I am at my typewriter, I don't hear or see my husband entering the room. At first my husband would call to me and, getting no response, would tap me on the shoulder. I would be startled, a response that would annoy him (we all have our sensitivities). My husband would explain that he disliked frightening me, and though I'd insist that I was not frightened, only startled, he would still be displeased. We found a solution: when he enters the room in which I am typing, he now turns off the light switch, which shuts off my typewriter. I'm no longer startled—just momentarily worried that my typewriter is broken. The flip of a switch has preserved household harmony.

A good way to attract the attention of a hearing-impaired person is to circle around that person until you are standing in his or her direct line of sight. Of course, this is not always practical—for example, I type at a table that is smack up against a wall.

Many problems in the home of a person with hearing impairment do not have simple solutions. "So," my friend says to me, "hearing impairment can really drive a wedge into a marriage."

"No," I answer, "the very working together for compatible solutions can make a marriage stronger and happier."

"I guess you have to give up pillow talk," my friend persists.

"Not at all," I tell her. "All you do is flip a switch, though I might add that sometimes less is more—less talk, more sex."

Chapter 3

Everyday Challenges

Morning to Night

From morning to night the challenge is there, although nighttime can almost be pleasant in the world of hearing impairment. Hearing aids removed, bedtime releases me from the creaking and settling of floorboards, from distant sirens that jar the nerves. Although, when they are close, sirens wail eerily like a hurt child, which is confusing because the wail of a hurt child is rarely heard at all.

With hearing aids removed, there is usually a peaceful environmental hum that helps me fall asleep, unless a superjet is approaching the nearby airport. Jets and thunder are indistinguishable. Many a night I have gotten up to close a window against the rain only to discover the night is moonlit and balmy. On other nights I have slept soundly through hail and heavy rain. So even nighttime separates the hearing world from the world of hearing impairment. Daytime shines a beacon on this separateness, exposing the constant daily challenge of impairment.

I am a writer but I am also a housewife, so for at least part of each day I am confronted with the challenges almost every person with hearing impairment faces.

Hearing aids are a must. Still, no matter how sophisticated, they are not a panacea. The severely damaged ear must make full partnership with the eyes. Even so, background noises cause tremendous hardship. The hum of voices and environmental sounds both inside and outside the home relegate the impaired, particularly the severely impaired, to a separate world.

Cursing the bad luck that has severely damaged your ears; worrying that your ears, if they are mildly or moderately impaired, will deteriorate to severe impairment; envying your dog when he hears the garbage truck that is still a mile away—these responses get you nowhere. Better to conclude that the affliction is part of nature's order, that you can train yourself to run with it as far as you choose by making its pieces fall into place. Impairment to the ears is a centipede with innumerable segments, so you need patience. Patience with yourself. Patience with others. It is too difficult to confront all aspects of this impairment at once. Better to take them one at a time.

Conquering Shopping

Through the window of the fish store, I see the dozen women and two men ahead of me. I pull a number and wait my turn. Other customers profit from this wait for numbers by examining fish soups and salads through huge glass refrigerator doors; selecting crackers, breads, or cocktail sauces from well-stocked shelves; or socializing. I remain attentive to the hanging numbers. Grace is only extended two numbers past the one you hold, a practice necessary to prevent customers from grabbing numbers, going elsewhere on the street to shop, and then returning with the expectation that they will be waited on immediately even though their number was called many digits back.

I watch patiently until I am two numbers from the one

I hold. A familiar-looking woman comes into the store, takes a number, and greets me effusively. We haven't seen each other for years. Immediately, I say, "Since we last met, I've lost much of my hearing." She answers, "We've all lost something along the way." We laugh and fill each other in on losses and gains of the past several years. When I check the number again, I see that the current number is more than two beyond my own; I have missed my turn. It is not easy for me to explain, amid the hum of customers' voices and the shuffling, cutting, and bagging by four men behind the counter, but I persist. Patiently but persistently.

My friend is helpful. She talks to the customer being served, who in turn explains to one of the men behind the counter. My number is reinstated and I am relieved that my 15-minute wait has not been in vain. I apologize to the man who takes my order. He remembers me as the woman who hears poorly but loves fish. Slowly, he describes the best method for preparing mahimahi. I lose some of his words, but because I am an old hand at fish I can improvise. It would not be fair for me to take too much of his time. He has already been kind enough to break the rule by serving me when my number was called many digits ago. I make a pact with him. Next time I will alert him that I am in the store, and he will make a special effort to prevent me from missing the call of my number. I make a pact with myself also: I shall always keep numbers in partial view no matter how tempting the distraction.

Next to the fish store is the Pottery & Gadgets Barn. Nothing in the store is a must, but I treat myself to a few minutes of browsing. A counter of mugs supporting a sign that announces a 50-percent reduction catches my eye; I can always use extra mugs. Unlike the fish store, business here is slow. Just one other woman, and she is edging toward the door, her browsing done.

I select several of the more colorful mugs, cautious not

to disturb a pyramid of sachets in their midst. The mugs are no bargain at their sticker price of six dollars, but at 50 percent off how can I resist! The lone salesperson stands nearby as I select mugs, commenting on the good price. "I love sales," I say and she mumbles back at me. I smile that sometimes foolish smile of a person with hearing impairment who doesn't quite understand what is said but feels it doesn't warrant the energy to explain the hearing problem or to educate the other in correct speech patterns.

When I put the four mugs I have chosen on the checkout counter, the saleswoman prepares to ring the sale on her cash register. "Just a minute," I say. "This is such a good deal at half price, I may as well make it a half dozen." Again I ignore her mumble and her surly expression and go back to the table of mugs for two more. I feel sorry for this woman whose business is so bad. I'm probably her big sale of the day, I tell myself.

When the saleswoman taps the cash register, I see the unit price per mug is six dollars. The grand total she is looking for is 36 dollars plus tax. I call the error to her attention and she mumbles.

"Sorry, I cannot understand you. My ears are very bad. Speak slowly and clearer please."

Now there is fire in her eyes, and what she says I do understand: "I keep telling you but you don't listen. The sale is for sachets. Not mugs."

"Well, that's the first thing you've said I can understand."

She mumbles.

"I explained my ears are very impaired."

She shouts a few words and I take a pencil and pad from the counter. "Never shout at people with hearing impairment. Your sign is as misleading as your voice. Please write."

She writes asking me if I want the mugs or not.

"I think not," I say. "But maybe we've both learned

something. Clear signs and clear speaking would have saved us both a lot of trouble. Mumbling is bad for your business. And it was *my* business to immediately explain my problem."

Supermarkets present different challenges to the hearing-impaired. In a crowded Pathmark I am looking for the aisle with paper napkins. Above the din I will hear nothing, so I tell the clerk, "I'm looking for paper napkins. My hearing is very impaired so please show me with your fingers what number aisle and please point the direction."

The young man raises five fingers and does better than point the direction. He leads me directly to the shelf I need. He more than compensates for the woman in the Pottery & Gadgets Barn, and in appreciation I thank him for his kindness and assistance.

In the produce department I do not have the good fortune to meet that helpful, well-spoken young man. Here all is hustle and bustle, with clerks ripping open cartons of fruit and vegetables to resupply dwindling stock. A bushel of corn contains only one shabby ear, and I would like to know if more corn will be brought to the floor. The young man I ask speaks little English. But he is pleasant, so I show him my hearing aids and tell him, "Just shake your head yes or no and I'll understand." "Ah, si, si," he grins and shakes his head. Again I am grateful and I thank him profusely. People with hearing impairment can pave the way for each other by showing gratitude to the helpful hearing.

There is one place to shop that lifts the spirits of people with hearing impairment: your neighborhood AT&T telephone store. I've been to several, so it is not by chance that people in my neighborhood AT&T store extend themselves as though they are specially trained to assist people with hearing impairment. Just announce your impairment in one of these stores, and you will be guided through a large assortment of assistive equipment with courtesy and expertise. The salesperson will let you use several phones, talking to you from another phone in the store, until you learn which instrument is best for you. Then you can take your selection home to try for 30 days to make certain it is good for you. For the person who has had difficulty communicating when shopping, a trip to an AT&T telephone store is a true morale booster.

Driving a Car

I have rules when I drive with others in my car. While seat belts are being buckled, I explain my situation in the driver's seat. Friends driving with me know about my impairment, so they accept my rules (which may have an unfair edge since I can talk to them freely whereas they cannot as freely talk to me).

"I need all my concentration for the road," I say, introducing rule number one. "If there's something you want a response to that I cannot understand without help from my eyes, it will have to wait until a traffic light." I continue with rule number two: "Please don't tap my shoulder for attention unless there is a danger I should be aware of." There is a tendency by hearing passengers to tap the shoulder of an impaired driver to get attention for nonessentials. In a car everything but the safety factor is nonessential. Actually, under any circumstance, tapping the shoulder of a person with hearing impairment is the least desirable method of getting attention.

Sirens always present a challenge to the hearing-impaired driver. The hearing driver can usually identify the direction the siren is coming from; the hearing-impaired driver often cannot. If there is a passenger seated next to me, I can ask that person to point to the siren's direction. I have trained myself to remain calm if I am alone and to watch other cars for clues, but mainly calmness does it. If the siren becomes louder, I know its direction will soon become visible. Hearing-impaired drivers generally keep themselves more alert than hearing drivers. Statistics show that drivers with hearing impairment have superior safety records.

I practice extreme courtesy on the road to minimize the need for other drivers to honk a horn at me. I can't understand the car radio or compact discs, so there is nothing to distract my attention from traffic. Safety, however, is not the only challenge to the hearing-impaired driver. Because vehicular noise makes it so difficult for me to understand people's voices, I must minimize the need to get directions. For all areas I drive through I keep a map; my glove compartment is a library of local maps. How simple it is to lose one's way on a winding suburban road! Of course, there are times I can't avoid talking to other drivers. If a lost driver is on a quiet road, I stop and listen carefully. The lost driver benefits from my impairment, which makes the glove compartment of my car a gallery of road maps. However, if the lost driver is in a car alongside mine on a major road, I can be of little or no assistance; I point to my ears to indicate my hearing problem.

If I am caught in a lengthy tie-up at a bridge or tunnel, I can't use my car radio for the traffic helicopter's advice. I am at the mercy of other drivers' strange voices under extremely noisy circumstances. For this challenge the Nasta Listenaider II always travels with me. This two- by four-inch unit is equipped for binaural reception through comfortable button headsets.

Usually, walking over to another car, explaining my impairment, and listening carefully is sufficient to get me understandable information. But there is comfort having my Listenaider available. I can hold this sensitive microphone near the driver I am asking for information. I rarely fail to get results.

The Listenaider offers another feature: a headphone with a 20-foot extension cord for use with TV or radio.

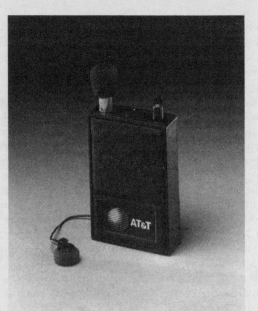

FIGURE 7. The Pocketalker

Impaired ears must be properly matched to assistive aids. I am unable to benefit from the TV and radio accessory, but the Listenaider serves me very well as a microphone and receptor for voices at close range. At its very low cost, it is a most attractive item in my wardrobe of assistive aids.

The Hearing-Impaired Passenger

Staying tuned to the conversation in a car is a challenge for the hearing-impaired passenger. The Pocketalker, similar in size and shape to the Listenaider, keeps me in touch with other passengers. The Pocketalker has two jacks: one for a microphone, one for an earphone. I remove the inch-long microphone, which is housed in a jack of the Pocketalker, attach it to the long cord provided with the unit, and hand the microphone to passengers seated either in front of me, behind me, or alongside me, that is, to anyone other than the driver.

I remove a hearing aid from one ear in order to use the earphone. The hearing aid in my other ear can pick up voices shut off from contact with the ear using the earphone. This gives me versatility. The microphone, with 12 feet of cord, enables me to interact with everyone in the car, except the driver. Passengers simply keep the microphone circulating.

Sitting alongside the driver, I can understand slow-moving lips from the side when there is adequate light. And because many hearing drivers make a practice of turning to the person seated next to them when they speak, I tell the person driving me that I do not want this usually appreciated courtesy of being faced. I feel I must explain that I do not need to be accommodated this way in a car. It is important for me to do this since at other times I have said, "Please face me when you speak."

When I am the passenger sitting up front, I can see the speech of the passengers behind me in my visor mirror unless it is dark out. Nighttime, the Pocketalker is my excellent assistive aid.

At the Dentist's

My annual dental checkup glues me to voicelessness. Only the probing of metal on enamel keeps me alert. If I am to speechread at all, it is the dentist's eyes I must read, since his mouth hides behind a protective surgical mask. Questions he asks whistle over me, making no sense. This is an intelligent man who knows about my hearing impairment (many times he has stored my hearing aids while taking X-rays). Still, he looks at me and what he sees is so normal, in all respects, that he tends to forget I cannot understand his speech through his surgical mask. When I come for my next appointment I will bring a gift: see-through clear plastic surgical masks.

The dentist talks on until I raise my hand and point to my ear. Then, elaborate with apologies, he removes his mask, and I am finally in a position to at least strain for what he is saying. Since I must keep my head still, I look, with difficulty, out of the very corner of my eye to catch a glimpse of speech. I cannot do this for very long and must raise my hand from time to time to request a breather as this very nice man keeps talking. He feels he must entertain me with stories about other writers he services, and although I am all curiosity my eyes can only take so much of a challenge during this long session of probing for cavities.

My dentist does accommodate my impairment, however, when accommodation is important: If he wants me to open my mouth wide, he raises his hand. If he wants me to hold my breath for an X-ray, he signals by turning the room light off and on. This language based on body movements and light can be practiced by all health care professionals.

Challenges That Surprise the Hearing

"You have to work pretty hard to keep current with the daily news," my husband tells me as we watch a telecaptioned TV sitting on our dinner table. This once chatty family time is now a dish of food and telecaption. Eating while reading captions has its drawbacks. My husband watches me wind spaghetti around my fork for an inordinate time. "Your dinner's getting cold," he says.

"So will the news be, if I stop watching."

My eyes do double time to read the fast-moving, frequently incorrect words, but I stay with it. What is the choice for a person with hearing impairment who yearns to remain knowledgeable about current world, national, and local events? News, on everyone's lips, is more urgent for me to feed on than spaghetti. There will be spots of tomato sauce on my sleeve or skirt, but that is the cost of daily living with hearing impairment.

Of course, every night is not spaghetti. When the menu allows, I practice what I have learned from my grandchildren: Let your fingers do the feeding. Still, spaghetti sauce spots or no, I am grateful to the telecaption on my table and to the television networks.

As I eat cool spaghetti, my husband tells me, "You're a good sport."

"People with hearing impairment better be," I answer.

Busy Thoroughfares

Walking in Manhattan with a friend, I concentrate on safety and miss much of the wider scene. My friend remains at my side, knowing that her voice, even in close range, is throttled by the din of vehicular traffic. Aware of my impediment, she knows I must have a clear view of her mouth; still, she can't restrain herself when there is a sight to be shared.

"Look at that," she says as we cross Madison Avenue. "Wait until we get across," I answer while I watch for cars turning from the cross street onto the avenue. I must also watch for pedestrians swinging packages and umbrellas that can trip me if I do not see them approaching. Surely, I will never hear them.

I feel I must apologize to my friend for not speechreading while we cross the street, "I need all my vision on this wide avenue. But I'll be with you soon." As if to emphasize my point, a poodle lopes alongside me and takes a swipe from his trainer. I catch this from the corner of my eye, or I would also be swiped with the training leash. Time was, crossing an avenue was a mindless stroll. Now it is a labor of eye-and-leg coordination. Appreciative of my problem, my good friend holds her observation until we are on the sidewalk. "What did you want me to see?" I ask. "Oh, just a weird hat some guy passing us was wearing." My friend's description will have to suffice.

Soon we are passing a construction site. Walking on streets where the racket of construction clobbers the ears, I turn my aids off. My friend cannot understand the peace I find walking with no hearing. I can continue to read her speech easily without the intrusion of howling machinery. I tell my friend, "Sometimes, deaf is better," and as I say this I am shocked because I have always berated hearing people who refer to people with hearing impairment as deaf.

I remember an incident in which I was referred to as deaf. Our heating oil supplier always rings my bell to alert me to shut off the heat while he fills the tank. He has a card that reads as follows: USE BELL. KNOCK ON WINDOWS, WALK AROUND THE HOUSE IF NECESSARY. CUSTOMER IS DEAF. "Never say deaf," I told him in fury when I saw the card he carries. "I'm hearing impaired. Never say deaf."

The word is not a pejorative. It is not an insult. It is not an embarrassment. People with severe hearing impairment are sisters and brothers to the profoundly deaf. It's just that we each have our separate identities and I want that understood. So I shock myself when I tell my friend about the peaceful state of making myself deaf in this thundering-noise-polluted city.

The shoe is on the other foot as my friend and I walk past the construction site. She hears nothing I say, but I can speechread her words. There is some danger in this deaf state I have made for myself as construction activity roars around us. My eyes are my only tools for recognizing a delivery cart speeding from behind. Children on skateboards are a menace. Pedestrians in running shoes can bowl me over. So I keep rotating my head as I walk, and I let my eyes do all the work. Of course, with my friend at my side there is comfort that she will tug me out of harm's way. Understanding my situation, she says, "Walking in the city is a chore for you." "It can be," I agree.

Soon we are on a block without construction and I tune myself back into the hearing world. If we walk leisurely I switch from my aids to my Listenaider. With the microphone clipped to my friend's jacket, we have a decent conversation. We are also a curiosity to some passersby.

I cannot worry about stepping into puddles or missing shop windows; people with hearing impairment must settle for a lesser view of the world. If we can speechread our walking companions, our day is a success; other sights are icing on the cake.

"So," my friend says when we get to our destination, "it should be easier for you inside the department store."

"Yes and no," I answer as I dodge a stockperson wheeling a cartload of merchandise. "Did you hear him coming?" I ask.

"Of course. Didn't you?"

"Not really. But I often feel vibrations or see shadows that alert me. A run-in with that heavy cart could really put me out of commission."

My friend stands closer to my side, aware of the many challenges that shape my ordinary day. "No wonder you get to bed so early and don't want phone calls at night."

"We all make our accommodations," I explain. "The need for extra bed rest is just one of the costs of daily living with hearing impairment. On the plus side is the telecaption TV in my bedroom."

"Are your favorite programs captioned?" she asks.

"No," I answer. "But you'd be amazed at how my tastes have changed to appreciate any program with those lovely word tags."

"So your eyes work hard day and night."

"Right. We people with hearing impairment get our money's worth from a good set of eyes."

Dealing with Servicepeople

I consider myself to be as competent as I was before hearing got hard and refuse to relinquish the responsibility of dealing with servicepeople. Those who have been servicing my home for many years are easier to work with than newcomers. So when the plumber rang my bell, I was disappointed to see a new, young face, especially one decorated with a walrus moustache, the bane of people with hearing impairment.

The new plumber toted a heavy tool chest and sounded as though he had a foreign accent, but my ears frequently detect an accent when in fact there is none. Only after a long and laborious explanation by me of how he must talk, he said, "So let's get to the problem."

"In here," I said, leading the way to the bathroom. He followed—too slowly, I thought, faulting his lack of ambition. "See," I said, showing him by flushing the toilet, "it needs some attention." Shaking his head, he muttered something unintelligible, which I took as a rebuke for bothering him when there was nothing wrong with the toilet (which did indeed flush properly in the presence of a plumber). "Look," I persisted, "sometimes it works and sometimes it doesn't." I flushed many times and the toilet performed to perfection. "I guess that's par for the course," I said. "The patient always feels better when the doctor arrives."

Seeing no humor in my remark, the young man removed his tool chest from the bathroom and sauntered back to the kitchen. "Believe me," I told him apologetically, "it's a toilet in need of repair."

Rubbing his nose to further compound the difficulty I was having speechreading through his troublesome walrus moustache, he demanded to know something I could not fathom. After many tries, I realized he wanted to know where my *bedroom* was. I felt a tug of terror. Why was it his business where my bedroom was located? Was this young man a rapist? Braving it, I decided to summon my Westie, Yogi, telling this rapist it was time for my dog's walk: "His toilet works and it's outside." I called for Yogi to come for a walk, an invitation that always brings him running. But not this time. I shook his leash, a maneuver guaranteed to get a response. Still, no Yogi. Had the rapist poisoned my dog? I needed to escape from my house, but the young man grabbed my arm, saying, "Lady, I don't have all day. You can do the job yourself." My adrenalin must really have been flowing for me to understand his words. From his tool chest he pulled a bottle of brown liquid. "Ah, Liquid Plumber," I quipped. "Just pour it in the toilet when it doesn't flush, right?"

"No," he replied, shaking his head. Then, taking a card from his wallet, he showed me that he was from the furniture repair service that had promised, weeks back, to send a person to repair the scratches on my bedroom unit the next time the man was in the neighborhood.

Red-faced, I led the furniture repairman to the bedroom. Passing the bathroom door, I heard the yelp; Yogi had been closed in there when I gave up on flushing the toilet for the "plumber."

Another serviceperson who presented a challenge was an exterminator. I am a respecter of nature and a friend to stray dogs and cats, squirrels, rabbits, butterflies. My husband had a bumper sticker made for me: I BRAKE FOR ANTS. So when our house was visited by a small rat or large mouse—we were never sure which—and the "visitor" stayed and stayed, eating pears ripening on our kitchen hutch and nibbling bars of soap on the sink, I phoned an exterminator. I was adamant as I left my message for the exterminating service: "No blood. No killing."

The day the exterminator arrived, he was quick to assure me—in a good voice, moving his mouth well—that he understood how I felt. "Not to worry," he said; he'd do a bloodless job for me. How I welcomed this decent man until he told me, "I have ten cats."

I lectured him on barbarism and cruelty and invited him to leave. "How dare you bring ten cats into my house to eat one poor little rat or mouse!" I told him I'd rather share my pears and soap and accused him of encouraging the worst instincts in the animal kingdom. I even accused him of setting a malignant example for innocent children. "Ten cats," I yelled, "to pounce on one little mouse. That's unconscionable!"

He had a pleasant smile as he patted my arm and explained, "Tin cat, lady. Tin cat." He showed me a little house that lures the creature safely inside. "You then take him to a woodsy area where you release him unharmed. See? Everybody's happy." He set the tin house at the base of my hutch, where the little creature climbed for his nightly feast of ripening fruit. I apologized to this very nice man, who said, "Not to worry. In my business I get used to all kind of ladies."

I promised myself that I'd be more cautious in the future. I didn't want my hearing problem to make me the kind of lady servicepeople have to get used to.

The Constant Challenge

"Ten cats" and "tin cats" look alike to the speech-reader and the troubled ear cannot differentiate between "ten" and "tin" except in the context of a sentence. Wasn't it logical for a person, unknowledgeable about tin cats, to think the exterminator said "ten cats?" There is nothing visible about the vowels *E* or *I* in the middle of a word. Another challenge might have been the confusion of *T* with *D*, both being formed by the tongue against the palate. Of course, "den cats" would have made no sense unless the conversation had been about a den filled with pets.

Every spoken word presents a challenge for people with hearing impairment. Every daily activity presents a challenge. Constant challenges make an ordinary day more difficult and far more tiring for the hearing-impaired than for the hearing. Being able to manage everyday challenges is also a most rewarding experience. Every day, we people with hearing impairment can thank family and friends who help. And we can thank ourselves.

Chapter 4

Psychological Impacts and Burdens

A wide range of hearing disorders separate the hearing-impaired, yet they share a commonality of experience in the hearing world and a commonality of emotional pain. In the following interview Dr. Wayne Weisner, a psychiatrist practicing in Manhasset, New York, talks about his own impairment in order to highlight the experiences and responses of most hearing-impaired people.

Dr. Wayne Weisner

Let me start with a few observations. People becoming hard-of-hearing usually don't want to admit it. They may not even recognize their impairment until others call it to their attention. And it is sometimes not called to their attention in a kind way.

They may be accused of "selective hearing." If they aren't told they are hearing selectively, they may be told, often by a mate, "You're tuning me out!" and, at the same time, may be told, "You should do something about your hearing." This puts a most unfortunate double burden on the person who is becoming impaired.

To understand the accusation of "selective hearing" leveled against the person becoming hearing impaired, it is important to know that when people become hard-of-hearing there are certain ranges that can give them difficulty. They don't lose all voice range at once. They may lose high range and be unable to understand women or children. They may lose low range and not hear men's voices clearly. So you see how unfair the accusation of selective hearing is. Though they *are* hearing selectively, it is not by choice. Their "tuning-out" is not psychological. And the unfairness is compounded because at the same time that hard-of-hearing people are being told they are "tuning-out" their mate, they are told they have a physical impairment and must do something about their hearing.

Sometimes there are accusations by hearing people to the hearing-impaired person, accusations such as "You're not paying attention. Concentrate!" or "You're shouting!" And when the hearing-impaired person speaks softly to avoid shouting, the accusation is often "Why are you whispering?" At times both accusations come from the same source. There is little awareness that a hearing-impaired person has difficulty modulating his or her voice. After all, the hearing-impaired cannot hear their own voices the way people with normal hearing can.

When I was in the army during the Korean War, I realized that I was losing hearing in one ear. Still, I had satisfactory hearing in the other ear, so I didn't worry. My hearing loss was not service-related, however. Later, when I took a residency in psychiatry, I had trouble hearing my supervisor and the medical director of the clinic. Their voices were too soft, and my second ear was also getting bad. My supervisor thought I was "selectively hearing" or "tuning out."

I considered making a change in my profession because of my hearing difficulty and discussed this with my wife. If my hearing got very bad, I thought I'd become a radiologist. But I solved the problem with hearing aids. I practiced psychiatry for 15 years with the impairment. The old psychiatrist joke—"Who's listening?"—may come to mind, but my patients always knew that I was listening. They would see me change a battery in my hearing aid, so they knew I had to be listening.

Of course, there were problems I encountered because of my hearing impairment. I would have to strain all day listening to patients to be sure I heard everything. Patients were cooperative when I asked them to speak up. But if they were particularly depressed, they would mumble or lower their voices again. By the end of the day I'd be very fatigued. I think fatigue is something most hearing-impaired people experience. Even with hearing aids, the impaired have to work very hard to understand what is being said. They must follow every lip movement. In other words, they cannot relax and have a nice, easy conversation as people with normal hearing can.

My kind of hearing impairment was able to be helped with a *stapes mobilization.* In this procedure, a doctor flips back the eardrum and moves back the three little bones in the middle ear. This gets rid of calcium deposits around the *stapes.* Then when sound hits the drum, the drum vibrates and transfers the sound to the stapes. My stapes mobilization was successful but, unfortunately, it did not last. After six months calcium redeposited, and there I was with hearing loss again. At that point the loss was more depressing than when I first began to notice it. I did finally get a *stapedectomy** operation in both ears.

---

* A stapedectomy is a procedure in which the stapes is surgically removed and replaced by a prosthesis. Dr. Weisner's ear disorder was otosclerosis, a conductive disorder (see next section of this chapter).

This raised my hearing to normal in both ears. How wonderful to hear birds chirping!

People with hearing impairment tend to get a little paranoid. And this is understandable. They think people are not talking loud enough on purpose or are mumbling deliberately so they cannot hear what is being said. And it is true that when people talk to a hearing-impaired person for a long period of time, they eventually tend to lower their voices because their voices get tired. So it is not imagination on the part of the hearing-impaired person. Another problem is that many people tend to shout at people with hearing impairment, and the hearing-impaired think these people are angry with them. Anger is associated with shouting. So paranoia is one of the problems.

Of course, it happens too that the person who is shouting at someone with hearing impairment also suffers. He too associates shouting with anger and in fact does tend to get angry as he shouts. The hearing-impaired person can be told that it is paranoid to think that the shouting hearing person is angry, and yet he may be correct that the person who is shouting is in fact feeling anger.

Another problem of a person with hearing impairment is loss of self-esteem. When I lost my hearing, I was conscious of this. An important part of you is not right. And wearing a hearing aid is not as fashionable as wearing glasses can be. Sunglasses may even be a fashion accessory, like jewelry. This is never true of hearing aids. They mark one as handicapped, and so there is a stigma attached to a hearing aid, just as years ago there was with glasses. When I was growing up, girls would rather stumble over obstacles than wear glasses. So today many people would rather stumble over words, would rather not hear correctly, than wear a hearing aid.

When I first became hard-of-hearing, I had a little box with a cord that would go up to the ear. Instead of just wearing the little box, I created a small sling, like a detective might use for a gun. I had my wife sew the sling into my shirt, where I could hide the hearing aid box. I was happier when hearing aids were improved so the entire apparatus could be worn behind the ear. But even that aid created problems: In the gym or in a pool or a sauna I couldn't wear my aid, which made meeting people a problem. I avoided talking with people because I couldn't hear them, which made me seem and feel unfriendly.

Conductive Hearing Loss: Otosclerosis

"Otosclerosis [is] a pathological condition of the bony labyrinth of the ear, in which there is formation of spongy bone (otospongiosis), especially in front of a posterior to the foot-plate of the stapes; it may cause bony ankylosis [stiffness] of the stapes, resulting in conductive hearing loss. Cochlear otosclerosis may also develop, resulting in sensorineural hearing loss."*

Early treatment for otosclerosis, a conductive hearing loss, is explained by Dr. Alan Austin Scheer of New York City as follows:

Before 1950 a *fenestration operation* was done, bypassing the eardrum. A window was made in the balance canals to let sound around the back door. It was a big operation and the success rate was only fair. This was replaced by the mobilization operation. This is what Dr. Sam Rosen first discovered. He accidentally loosened a little bone—the stapes—and sound came through. That was when I started to get involved. I did many mobilization operations, but in seven out of ten cases, where the bone was too locked and wouldn't loosen up, we would break the bone. One out of three we were able to loosen

* From *Dorland's Illustrated Medical Dictionary,* 27th ed., s.v. "otosclerosis."

sufficiently to let sound come through. And of the one out of three patients who heard, 70 percent lost hearing again because the bone tightened up. Then we began to remove the stapes and replace it. John Shea made the major breakthrough of removing the stapes. The prosthesis replacement, which looks like Teflon, is a stainless steel piece that hooks onto the incus and transmits sound to the inner ear. The stapedectomy procedure has not really changed since 1962. It is a very predictable procedure but not foolproof.

In November 1991 Dr. Scheer explained a recent improvement he developed:

"The change in the procedure, is the fact that a smaller piece of the *footplate* [a portion of the stapes] is removed, lessening the possibilities of inner ear reaction—vertigo, and possible further loss of hearing. The Scheer Teflon wire prosthesis has proved to be most effective, rather than the solid Teflon prosthesis."

The Psychological Burden

The Gallaudet Encyclopedia of Deaf People and Deafness (Van Cleve, 1987) deals thoughtfully with the psychological burden of everyday challenges. The following section, reproduced with permission from McGraw-Hill, publisher of the *Gallaudet Encyclopedia,* was written by Howard E. Stone, a former executive director of Self Help for Hard of Hearing People, Inc. (SHHH).

Hard-of-Hearing

The psychology of people who are hard-of-hearing differs significantly from that of deaf people. Hard-of-hearing is used here to describe persons who have postlingually acquired hearing losses ranging from mild to profound but who can still benefit from amplification. Their speech is adequate for communication, and they use, however imperfectly, the auditory mode to receive communications. This invisible condition of diminished hearing, without external evidence such as signing, places such people in limbo. They do not belong to deaf communities, and they are usually estranged from the hearing community of which they had been a part. Uncertainty, anxiety, and the development of chronic stress produce adverse perceptions that perpetuate a vicious cycle. Fatigue, caused by the strain of concentrated listening and lipreading, reduces the hard-of-hearing person's physical and mental capability to function and to cope.

As people lose their hearing, things seem to change for them, and for those around them. Misperceptions of each other, fueled by interactions often caused by ignorance, evolve. Communication breaks down. Isolation—a feeling of being alone, even in the middle of a crowd—develops the trend toward withdrawal. Perceived rejection sets in, accompanied by poor self-esteem. The process of socialization gradually shuts down.

Stress Factor

Illness and disease often occur in individuals who have experienced a series of psychologically stressful events. Regardless of age, stress and one's reaction to it appears to be the critical factor. The loss, even partial, of the sense of hearing—upon which most interpersonal communications depend—may be described as a chronic stressor. It is a major life loss. The effort for a hard-of-hearing person to stay in effective communication requires tremendous physical and emotional energy beyond that required normally by a hearing person. The breakdown of communications causes intense stress. Hard-of-hearing people live with this stress constantly. Such unrelenting pressure, involving biological and psychological reaction to threatening situations in which people find themselves at a disadvantage, causes changes in behavior. The complexity of the task of adjustment by persons who lose hearing, and the effects on the people with whom they live, has never been fully appreciated.

Chronic stress is not an inevitable cause of psychological problems. Much depends upon how the stressor (hearing loss) is perceived and what the response to it is. When a major life crisis is seen as a challenge, coping is within reach. When the same life event is perceived as a crushing blow, helplessness and depression negate effective coping. A positive attitude minimizes the scope of the problem and enhances motivation to do something about it. Once the mind grasps the need for change or a readjustment and is open to information on how best to effect such change, there is a good chance for successful handling of the problem. Not that hearing can be restored or corrected (most hearing losses cannot), but tolerance, gained through acquiring skills which help one adapt to new circumstances, is a constructive response to stress.

Complications

While little is known about their adjustment, it is known that persons with acquired hearing loss have adjustment problems that are sometimes severe. Everywhere such people turn, they have a communication problem— on the street, in school, at the dinner table, in bed, on the job, in the doctor's office, in the market, on the phone, watching television, at the theater.

Every day, every endeavor is a fresh reason for anxiety. Failure is always imminent. Frustration is endless. Anger and resentment may be repressed or expressed in antisocial behavior. Tension and anxiety contribute to fatigue that further impedes communication. The inability of some people to project their voices, the unwillingness of many hearing people to make a special effort, to spend the extra time, lead hearing-impaired people to feel tentative, left out, suspicious, lonely, isolated, uninteresting, devalued, and depressed.

This is true of children, teen-agers, and young adults. It is especially true of middle-aged and elderly people who grew up with normal hearing and have no experience coping with an acquired hearing disability. They try the patience of family and friends. They do not want to ask people to repeat or to shout so they stay home more often, and become more withdrawn. The unaccustomed isolation leads to depression.

Perception

Coping means acceptance of hearing loss, reduced access to social situations, and the wearing of a hearing aid. The hearing aid is expected to correct the situation to a significant degree. Family members will then strike a balance between support and dominance so that the hearing-impaired person can be effective, independent, and a participant in family life.

It almost never works that way. Studies of persons with acquired hearing loss, particularly in the United Kingdom, point to a lack of coping and to inappropriate adjustment, which lead to dissatisfaction on the part of the individual.

The degree to which a person can tolerate the reduced and varying extent of access to information will determine the degree of adjustment. If the person is to achieve a satisfactory level of communication, every encounter between hearing and hard-of-hearing persons requires that communications contracts be negotiated with patience and sensitivity. In the choice between changing one's life style to increase control or withdrawing from those areas of previous life style that now threaten independence and control, the latter seems more likely.

Adjustment Phases

To facilitate understanding of the forces at play when hearing loss occurs, the three phases through which a person might travel in the process of adjustment should be examined. These are described below.

Phase I. The first phase is the period before the person acknowledges hearing loss and seeks help. The extent of Phase I varies from days to years. Although conscious realization of hearing impairment may take a long time, adjustment is in progress. Estimates indicate that three-fourths of those with acquired hearing loss are in this phase at any given time. These are people who have not sought professional help with their problem. A common response in this phase is to increase control of loudness (turn up the television, radio, and stereo) and to increase use of social and physical means to enhance intensity of information sought (sit closer to the speaker at meetings, increase concentration, make frequent requests for repetition). The hearing person's reaction to such action includes complaints about loudness, nonverbal acts such as hands over ears, and refusal to repeat—"It isn't important." The resulting alternatives are either a reduced level of loudness or an alienation of others. In either case, the hearing-impaired person is on the defensive and has to adjust to the lesser of two evils.

As these situations occur more frequently, the hearing-impaired person moves closer to seeking help, often at the insistence of family members; accelerates the process of aggressive and antisocial behavior; or withdraws from normal social activities. The individual exists in a twilight zone, unable to hear in the sunlit world of sound, yet not enveloped in a night of silence; ambiguity becomes the problem. Phase I, combined with aging, poses an increasingly difficult problem for the hearing-impaired person which all too often has resulted in institutionalization.

Phase II. The diagnosis and referral phase is normally of short duration, but it is one of great anxiety. The diagnosis of hearing loss (often progressive) opens many possibilities for the future: total deafness, loss of job, embarrassment, stigma, loss of independence, rejection by family and friends. The person is usually less focused on the physical aspects of hearing loss than on the social, economic, and personal costs of the new circumstances. How the doctor, audiologist, hearing aid specialist, family, and friends perform in this phase can be crucial to the hearing-impaired person's ultimate adjustment. The degree and direction of adjustment in Phase I also has bearing on where the hearing-impaired person will go from here. Information can help. A clear understanding of what is and what is not happening to the person can contribute to a positive reaction. Awareness that there are many others in similar circumstances and actually meeting some of the problems is very useful.

Phase III. Most of the literature of acquired hearing loss falls into this category—adjustment to diagnosed hearing loss. Whatever support came from family and friends in the previous two phases must now be replaced by long-term commitment. This becomes as difficult for them as for the hearing-impaired person because misunderstandings develop easily. The hearing-impaired person feels the family does not understand the problem, and the family feels the person is not accepting the hearing loss, and is not adjusting properly. For the small percentage who use hearing aids successfully, the struggle to maintain some degree of control in interpersonal relationships is enhanced, but tension is usually present and adjustment comes to mean dealing with diminished control.

Support Structure for Adjustment

One need not become psychologically debilitated or even chronically unhappy as a result of hearing loss. But the requirements for successful adjustment are not within the sole control of the individual. The response to hearing loss is conditioned by significant others and members of the hearing health delivery system. Acquisition of information about hearing loss, learning new skills in communication, associating with others who are in similar circumstances all contribute to potential for successful handling of the problems that hearing loss poses.

Chapter 5

Dropping Out and Returning

Because hearing impairment is invisible, it is frequently unnoticed by the hearing community. At times it is misinterpreted. The impaired person who sits quietly, understanding nothing in a group conversation, may be considered dull, dim-witted, antisocial, or a snob to be ignored.

Awareness of the disability by the hearing community often comes in partnership with embarrassment, and sometimes with deep feelings of helplessness or an intense desire to be of assistance. Unfortunately, many in the hearing community do not know how to be of assistance.

Sometimes the hearing will be impatient or exasperated with futile attempts to make themselves understood, and they will simply withdraw from people with hearing impairment.

Negative responses by the hearing community are often cries of frustration or despair because a loved one is separated—set adrift, in a sense—from the world of hearing persons. The separation, the drifting away, can be difficult for the hearing to believe because in all other respects people with hearing impairment are so normal. As a result, skepticism may be added to frustration and despair. Then too everyone has the fear that if this can happen to a loved one—a sister, brother, friend—"it can happen to me!" Burdened this way, it is difficult for the hearing to respond positively.

Very few people with hearing impairment have not experienced negative responses by the hearing community. Some have not had the good fortune to meet knowledgeably helpful hearing people, and they choose to withdraw before they are once again withdrawn from. They keep to themselves within the sea of noise, the chatter and laughter, in the world of the hearing.

Of course, there are those in the hearing community who are instinctively sensitive to the hearing-impaired, who know just how to talk and how to assist when others do not make themselves understood. People with hearing impairment are grateful to these natural friends and hope to extend their sensitive knowledge to the rest of the hearing community.

Some people learn to manage their hearing impairment with little difficulty, particularly those with only mild impairment. As impairment progresses to moderate and then severe, the management becomes more difficult. When impairment becomes severe, many become estranged from the hearing community. They drop out and blame their isolation on everyone but themselves.

Profile of a Dropout

I met Cynthia at a "meet your candidate" social. Ours is a small village, so I knew who Cynthia was. Most everyone in our village knew who she was—the mother of twin boys, the stars of the junior high's tennis team. But until that social, Cynthia and I had had no direct contact.

We were seated side by side on plushy ottomans, and I introduced myself. Cynthia smiled broadly. Her husband, standing several feet away, called out to me, "She doesn't hear a thing you're saying." His remark startled me— sickened me, actually—because one of my rigid arrangements with my husband makes it off-limits for him to announce my impairment for me. I make my own announcements. People with hearing impairment have disabled ears, but in all other ways they are normal people. When announcements are made for them, they feel demeaned.

Cynthia's broad smile, an almost artificial grin, as she sat next to me either hearing or partially hearing her husband (at the very least she was aware that he was talking to me about her) made her feel like a child. She told me this the next morning as we started to become good friends. "Sometimes," she said, "I feel as though people think I'm retarded. You're the only one I can speak to like this. It's too upsetting to discuss with anyone else."

"Even your husband?" I asked.

"Especially my husband," she answered, tears welling in her eyes.

In a group Cynthia would sit with a broad, frozen smile, not typical of the expressive face I'd see on the tennis court when she'd play with her twin sons and her husband and certainly not typical of her face when we had our long one-on-one talks, which began the morning after the "meet your candidate" social.

I think Cynthia changed her regular jogging route that morning. I had never noticed her passing my house before, and during breakfast I always glance up from the newspaper to watch joggers and walkers. Cynthia would have made an impression because she, unlike the other joggers passing my house each morning, wasn't quite dressed for the act: what was missing was a Walkman headphone, something most joggers wear to keep tedium out of the jog. At breakfast each morning I would give this headgear a lot of thought, envying the hearing who could add a little music, a talk show, news, or maybe even the chapter of a novel to their exercise. How I'd speculate on all the wonders they were tuned in to!

Were these hearing joggers aware of their good fortune? Probably not. Didn't I too once take hearing for granted? Did I ever congratulate myself on my luck in being able to listen to the radio while driving the car or preparing dinner? Of course not. Good hearing was my born right. I never gave it a second thought—until I lost it.

Unadorned by a Walkman, Cynthia was straining to see past an overgrown shrub that screened the breakfast room's bay window from the road. She slowed down almost to a crawl, and I got the feeling she was a fellow hearing-impaired in trouble, or at least in need of communication.

At the foot of my driveway our solid friendship began. We walked slowly so we could see each other's mouths, and we talked as though we had known each other all our lives. Sun had begun to warm the icy streets to slush, and my rubber boots and Cynthia's jogging shoes made extraordinary sounds. People with hearing impairment who were born into the hearing world associate sounds with old experiences that would hardly make sense to the hearing. For example, each time Cynthia's shoes smashed lumps of snow, she was reminded of how her twins, when they were five or six, would pretend to be dogs and bark at each other. As for me, the sound of boots on snow was window shades being rolled up and down.

When we finished comparing the way we heard sloshing noises, Cynthia told me about an evening when she and her husband went to his brother's apartment for dinner. She sat alone with the men for ten or fifteen minutes while her sister-in-law put the children to bed. "It felt like an hour," Cynthia said, "because neither my husband nor brother-in-law looked in my direction as they talked. At one point my brother-in-law glanced at me and said,

'You're awful quiet this evening.' I saw red! I said, 'I can't have a conversation by myself. You're both hiding your lips from me.' Then there was terrible quiet and embarrassment all around. I was sorry I came down so hard on them but they of all people should know better.''

I told Cynthia, ''I can't count the times I've thought people should know better. Thoughtlessness is probably more common than the common cold. And, I'm sure, in many ways we're also guilty of thoughtlessness. It just seems more unforgivable, to those of us with hearing impairment, when a relative or husband is thoughtless. The other evening my husband answered a phone call that happened to be from someone who was getting information for me about a hearing-impaired actor I want to interview. I was at the back of the house getting dressed, and we were running short of time for an appointment in the city. Without consulting me, my husband asked if I could return the phone call in the morning. In my hearing days he'd have called to me in another part of the house. Of course, this is impossible now, and in the interest of saving time he spoke for me. It so happens that that was one call I'd have made time for. I had trouble composing myself to ask, with a fairly civil tongue, that he never do that again. Unfortunately, we people with hearing impairment are too easily offended.'' I told Cynthia, ''Before we were impaired, we probably did our share of mishandling hearing-impaired people. Hearing impairment may be the most mishandled impairment.''

''That's true,'' she agreed. ''If we were blind, people would be at our side to help us cross streets. They'd lead us. Why can't they lead us with careful speech?''

I told Cynthia, ''There is something I usually do when people tend to forget my impairment. I hate to sound critical, so I bend the facts a bit and say, 'You really move your mouth very well. If you could just face me more directly— the light here is quite poor.' I try getting my point across without making them feel guilty.''

Walking on a little-traveled suburban street, people with hearing impairment cannot be as relaxed as hearing walkers can be. Often, they will not hear a car coming from behind and will only be aware of it once it has passed. So Cynthia and I walked against traffic, our attention divided between watching each other's mouth and taking safety precautions, that is, eyes partially on the road, antennae alert for cyclists or runners who might come from the rear (I think people with hearing impairment develop eyes at the back of their head!).

Because ours is a small village, drivers and walkers frequently acknowledge each other even if they are not acquainted. During our first long walk and talk, a car stopped. A young woman jumped out to hug Cynthia, who hunched into herself and made no introduction. I stood by, embarrassed. This was obviously a one sided friendship. The young woman extended a hand to me, explaining that she was Cynthia's neighbor.

I tried losing myself in the glistening snowscape, patches so paper thin on lawns you could see down to spring-green. The sun was strong and I watched the last of winter melting into the culvert while the young woman expressed joy at seeing Cynthia and chagrin that they hadn't gotten together for such a long time. She spoke clearly and I understood most words though I purposely averted my eyes. Cynthia made no response. The young woman told Cynthia she didn't know what had happened between them and Cynthia remained quiet. Finally, the young woman got back into her car, and my peripheral vision caught her limp wave. Cynthia's face was glued to the ground.

"She's a social climber," Cynthia told me. "We used to be best friends. Before, that is." Cynthia's severe hearing impairment was recent. No one actually knew what made her very mild hearing problem so severe—although as our friendship grew and as Cynthia talked about the medication her doctor had given her for elevated blood pressure, we both began to have suspicions.

Cynthia had been a teacher before her impairment became severe, and she was quite bitter that she'd had to give it up. She was also bitter about her social-climbing neighbor. "So wasn't she a social climber when you were best friends?" I asked Cynthia.

"I suppose. But I was the one she was out to cultivate. I guess I was flattered. It's my own fault. I should have known a person like that wasn't worthwhile. I mean, she was dying to play tennis with me. And what a bum she was. But I rallied with her when she couldn't get into a game with other women. I helped her develop a fair game. In addition, one of her kids was in my class, so she really worked at cultivating my friendship. I don't know what I ever saw in her, but we were best friends for several years. Our husbands got on well too. They had a regular poker game; in fact, they still do. She really worked at developing a couple-to-couple friendship. My husband is quite a comedian. He's got such a repertoire of jokes he could be a pro, if he gave up dentistry. And he plays the piano, so he's always the life of the party."

Cynthia was breathless with the need to complain about her social-climbing neighbor. "As couples, we'd go to the theater regularly. To neighborhood movies and restaurants. We were an inseparable foursome. We joined a Great Books group, and weekends we'd go to readings at the 92nd Street Y. Then this thing happened to me."

"There are still things you could do together."

"Of course. But she didn't go out of her way one bit. I mean, considering how decent I'd been to her. I helped her get started with a tennis group. Introduced her to all my friends. Then my hearing went. I couldn't enjoy the book group anymore. Most theater was out for me. Movies, except for foreign films, were impossible."

"Well, you couldn't expect her to give up films, theater, and book groups."

"I didn't expect that. But I did expect her to put herself out a little. I mean, one day I was real down. I asked if she and her husband would go to dinner. She said they were going to dinner with two other couples and she knew I wouldn't enjoy joining them because I couldn't hear in restaurants with large groups. I was outraged. How many times I had included her with other couples when she had nothing to do!"

"How did your husband react?" I asked.

"Well, naturally, he thought it very unkind of her. But that didn't interfere with the big greeting he still gives her. He thinks I'm too sensitive. He laughs everything off. Tells me to lighten up."

For our next walk and talk I was prepared with my Pocketalker, explaining that Cynthia should use the receiver and I would talk into the microphone. She was stunned at the clarity with which she heard my words. I suggested she try it at the book group she used to go to with her social-climbing neighbor.

"I'm not big on second-time-arounds," she said. "I mean I have to protect myself from being hurt a second time. That's why I'm letting my husband cover the school conference tonight. I'm not repeating the fall conference with this teacher. She talked to my husband the entire conference, as though I were a piece of furniture. Don't forget I'm—or should I say *was*—a teacher too, so I know the routine. I also know my boys are high achievers, so the interview is merely a pleasantry. And, true, the room was noisy and it was difficult for me to understand what was being said. Still, she could have tried harder."

"Did you, when you were a teacher?"

"Did I what?"

"Always try harder. Didn't you ever talk with two parents and direct your attention to the one who was most responsive? Did you always know the condition of the less responsive parent's ears?"

Cynthia understood what I was saying, but I wasn't

sure she was about to give this teacher a second chance. I decided that Cynthia, a young woman who had so much— an athletic, vigorous husband who looked like Robert Redford and was the life of the party, twin boys who starred on tennis courts and in classrooms—was the saddest and loneliest woman in our village.

My new friend Cynthia was a perfect candidate for Self Help for Hard of Hearing People, Inc. (SHHH). I invited her to come with me to the next meeting of the local SHHH group.

Dropping Back In

A hospital has given SHHH a home. The meeting Cynthia attends with me is held in a room that is bare except for a circle of plain wood chairs. Twenty-five of us sit in this spare ambience. A man is speaking into a microphone.

Cynthia tells me, "I can't hear a thing." "Turn your hearing aids to the T position," I explain. Her face brightens. This very ordinary room is made magical by a wire loop surrounding the chairs. The area loop is 100 watts of amplifying power delivered through flat wire; it can be tucked under carpeting or placed around floor molding with adhesive clips. The loop works in conjunction with hearing aids set on their T (telephone) position. The system eliminates background noise interference and brings voices to the impaired ear with such clarity that the impaired ear has almost normal comprehension or discrimination.

Since her impairment, this is the first public meeting at which Cynthia has been able to understand what is being said. Hungrily, she and I hang on to each word. I think about the response when I mention my impairment to people in the hearing world: "Don't worry. Most of what is said is usually nonsense anyway." Only the hearing

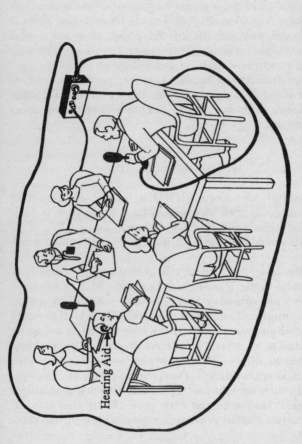

FIGURE 8. An audio loop system. (Reproduced by permission of the artist Frank Furio and Advocates for Better Communication, League for the Hard of Hearing.)

think this way. Nonsense, inanities, banalities, non sequiturs—once I became impaired, I wanted to hear all of them. I suppose what I really wanted was to be able to make my own choice of what to listen to and what to tune out. With the loop I and the other SHHH members have that option—though as I look around the room it is clear no one exercises the option to tune out.

Before the guest speaker arrives, our chairperson discusses the Americans with Disabilities Act (ADA)—recent legislation that will enable the lives of people with hearing impairment to be enriched. She explains it will be up to us to request facilities to which we are entitled. We must alert hotels that we require certain assistive devices like telephones with volume control, and we must request the workplace to supply us with special telephones—either a phone with volume control or a text telephone (TTY). Then the chairperson encourages discussion of hearing-related experiences. The woman at my right borrows the microphone. "There are many ways," she says, "the community could make hearing possible for us. I went to see my son in a school play today. See is a precise description: I sat as close as I could and still heard nothing. How simple it would have been for them to have the same kind of loop we have in this room around one row of chairs in the school auditorium. Not only would they accommodate hearing-impaired parents like me but there are probably schoolchildren who would benefit from a loop also. I'm going to speak to the Parents' Group about raising the $700 for a loop."

A man takes the microphone to complain that his wife speaks so slowly to him, pausing between each word. He says, "It's as though she's trying to humiliate me."

Another man says, "That's better than my wife. Mine sounds like an engine racing. Sometimes I think she doesn't want me to understand what she's saying."

A woman confides, "You really learn a lot about your mate when your hearing goes. But, really, you should have learned about them before your hearing went. I used to keep my radio on WINS when I was preparing dinner. My husband used to complain that I was ridiculous listening to the same news over and over. It really rankled me that he was bothered by my choice of diversion while I did boring household chores. But, thinking back, it really makes me angry. It's as though he put a hex on me because now my ears are so bad I can't listen to the radio at all. I know it's foolish of me to feel this way and I'm sure he meant nothing mean by his criticism, but it does make you think about your own behavior, about being kinder and less critical of people. You just don't know when you're pressing a sensitive nerve or when your criticism will backfire."

A woman with severe hearing impairment tells about an experience she had that morning that still has her edgy. She was shopping, and when she returned to her car the motor was dead. She went to the lobby of a department store to call the AAA, but not one phone in the bank of telephones was equipped with volume control for the benefit of people with hearing impairment. She stood crying near the bank of useless phones until finally some stranger made the call for her.

Members of our local SHHH group are very sympathetic and almost everyone wants to relate a nightmarish experience about needing a phone and not finding one with volume control.

A woman with mild to moderate impairment tells about an experience at the office in which she works. At times she must handle the telephone. Usually, she has no difficulty, but one day a call came in from a person with a whispery voice. Her request that the caller please repeat herself or himself—she wasn't even sure of the person's gender—was rebuffed with an impatient sigh, more whispers, and a slammed receiver.

The chairperson had recommendations: "Turn a whisperer over to someone else in the office who can determine if the problem is with the caller or with the connection. If this is not feasible, take an assertive stance. Ask questions like 'Are you calling to place an order?' or 'Are you calling with a complaint?' These questions may enable you to put a whisperer through to the proper department."

The room becomes lively with others who have had similar experiences. A man tells about a department manager who mumbles directives, leaving him intimidated and worried about losing his job. The chairperson says, "The fault is often the mumbler's. Mumbling can be a cover for their not having a clear idea of what they want to assign an employee. Just ask the department manager to please repeat the confusing part of the assignment. Possibly, the hearing people you work with experience the same difficulty. A competent manager should want to give assignments with clarity and good voice."

The microphone passes quickly from hand to hand. One man says his problem is the result of learning to speechread so proficiently that his family and friends tend to forget he is impaired and as a result revert to the old habit of fast-paced speech.

Cynthia is thoroughly enjoying this rap session. She asks for the microphone and describes her bitterness when her ears became severely impaired. "My husband took me to an ear specialist, who directed himself only to my husband. It was as though I were an infant or a retarded child. I've had other bad experiences too with people who should know better. My twins' teachers, for example. The minute my husband tells them I'm hearing impaired, they act as though I've dissolved. Doctors and teachers have had lots of schooling, but what they really need is instruction in good manners. That's what it's all about. Good manners."

Several members grab for the microphone to tell

Cynthia she must not let her husband make the announcement about her impairment. One woman explains that Cynthia puts herself in the position of being immature when she does not explain her own impairment and that from then on a new relationship may go downhill.

When Cynthia and I take our next walk, I will pursue the importance of making your own announcement and will tell her about my unfortunate experience before I insisted that my husband must always leave the telling to me.

The guest speaker this evening is a teacher at a school for the deaf. She brings with her a folder filled with illustrations of the hand positions of the sign alphabet, which she distributes. She demonstrates the alphabet and suggests we all learn it. She thinks it a fine idea for our mates

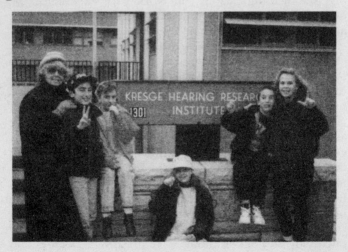

FIGURE 9. At the Kresge Hearing Research Institute, University of Michigan Medical School: the author and (from left to right) Adam, Anna, Rebecca, Andrew and Virginia, all using the manual alphabet. (Photo by A. Kadushin)

to learn it as well. Many words are impossible to understand because it is so difficult to speechread the beginning of the word, that is, the first letter. The letter *C,* for example, hides way back in the throat. If someone can sign that letter *C,* understanding the word will be much easier for the impaired person.

This SHHH meeting has helped establish Cynthia on the road to taking charge of her impairment. And it has positioned all of us on the road to better communication with both the hearing world and with the deaf community.

Cynthia folds her illustration of the sign alphabet carefully. She will encourage her husband and her twin sons to learn it with her. I will encourage my husband to learn it also.

Driving home from the SHHH meeting, I tell Cynthia why my husband has already learned a few manual or sign letters: At dinner one evening my husband told me he met the daughter of an old friend of mine. "She's a loner," I heard him say. I responded, "How do you know?" Realizing I had not heard correctly, he repeated the word, which I then heard as "lonesome." He laughed and tried again. When people with hearing impairment miss the first few guesses, the tendency can be to reach for the correct word. "Are you telling me she's loose?" I asked. "I wouldn't know," he replied, laughing too hard to continue eating. My next guess was "loaded." "Very rich?" I asked. Now his look was pure bewilderment. "Don't tell me she was loaded with liquor," I said.

"Just a minute, sweetheart," he said getting up from the table for pencil and paper.

"Ah, she's a *clone* of her mother. But of course, she always was."

That troublesome *C* when it sounds like a *K.* A letter unseen is the bane of people with hearing impairment. How simple with the manual alphabet (Figure 10). *C* is an easy letter for the hearing to learn. Easy even for very young children. It is merely a cup on end. When my granddaughter Virginia Louise was in second grade, her teacher taught the class the manual alphabet. Oh, the many happy hours Virginia Louise and I have spent using our fingers to spell secrets to each other!

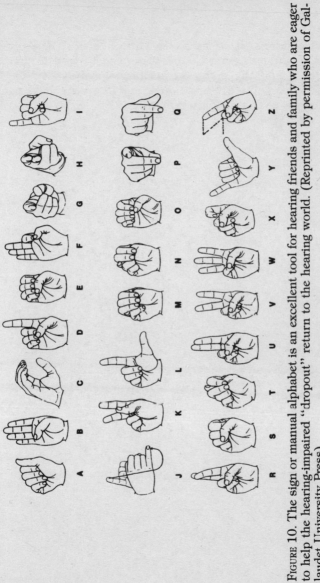

FIGURE 10. The sign or manual alphabet is an excellent tool for hearing friends and family who are eager to help the hearing-impaired "dropout" return to the hearing world. (Reprinted by permission of Gallaudet University Press)

Chapter 6

Interacting from Soup to Nuts

Dinner—Sweet and Sour

At many functions catered by my husband's company I sit with people I am meeting for the first time. While my husband is bullish or bearish at a far table, I am expected to interact congenially at my table. Although I am not shy about announcing my impairment to strangers, I sometimes do not have this opportunity before a conversation is under way between my table partners, that is, the guests to my immediate left and right, and the guest on the other side of them. This was the situation one evening during the season newspapers were headlining the British author Salman Rushdie and the Iranian death threat against him.

Nowhere in that room was there a rug to dim the laughter and the multitude of voices, making it impossible for my severely impaired ears to comprehend a word. Nor could I see past the head of my immediate partners, bent attentively to the guest on their other side, to make sense of the fast-moving lips. Through hot appetizer and cold soup I communed with a centerpiece of wildflowers and felt glum.

While wine to accompany the entree was being poured, I concentrated on a young woman across the table. Her mouth moved well and I could see that she and the men on either side of her were evaluating hostile takeovers. I felt myself coming alive, merging with the hearing world. The men seated next to me lost their silent partner.

It was a strain to see past the flower arrangement to the young woman's lips. I could not do this and eat at the same time, but I preferred to use my mouth for activity other than chewing. I was hungry for an opportunity to speak during the three-way conversation about takeovers, though I worried about breaking in with a contribution that had already been hashed and rehashed. I watched carefully, waiting to have my say. But I waited too long. On the young woman's lips I could see the conversation had changed from poison pills to poisoned apples.

The men on either side of the young woman became quite animated, frequently speaking at once, making it impossible for a speechreading person to follow them. But even when they spoke singly, most of their words were chewed along with their food and I was lost. I waited for the young woman to enter the apple pesticide battle, but she was merely nodding and eating. My patience was finally rewarded. I could discern the words "Red Delicious" and "Macintosh." I got no handle on other things the men were saying but I assumed they were angry because their favorite apples were being poisoned.

Here was my opportunity to add humor to this very heavy conversation. I had no worry that I would be repeating what had already been said. I would tell my personal anecdote. "Two years ago," I called across the table, "we planted a Red Delicious and a Macintosh tree. The following spring we got little hard knots of fruit that turned out to be quince."

The young woman and her partners listened with polite, quiet attention. I decided to embellish the story to get a laugh, but the woman smiled pleasantly and then talked with her partners. I saw on her well-paced lips that apple pesticides were no longer the topic. It was Rushdie and his wife, Maggie, the men were discussing when I intruded my story about buying mislabeled trees. When I thought apples were the subject, I saw "Red Delicious" on the lips of the man saying "Rushdie" and "Macintosh" on the lips of the man saying "Maggie." It is easy for a person with hearing impairment to see what she thinks she should be seeing.

Through dessert and coffee that evening I remained mute and embarrassed. But to the next business function catered by my husband's company I came equipped with an assistive aid, which I placed on the table in front of me. It was unnecessary for me to interrupt conversations of dinner partners to explain my impairment. The little box did it for me. It became an object of great interest, even getting more of a play than junk bonds and leveraged buyouts.

The Little Box on the Table

The two components of the Williams Sound Personal FM System, a wireless listening system, are similar in size and shape to the Pocketalker and the Listenaider. Like the Listenaider, the Williams system is binaural. The binaural earphones used with the receiver can be customized by an audiologist to snap into the listener's personal ear molds. This adapting gives the listener the kind of comfortable access to sound he or she gets from hearing aids. The wireless receiver can be kept in the listener's pocket. Because the system is wireless, there is no interference or blockage between the listener and the speaker using the wireless transmitter.

A small microphone with a lapel clip plugs into the transmitter, which the speaker can keep in a shirt or blouse pocket. With the microphone at a reasonable distance from the mouth, the speaker's words are relayed clearly to the listener.

When there is group conversation, such as when guests are seated around a dining table, the microphone and transmitter can sit on the table, giving the listener access to several speakers. The little box on a dinner table should be protected from table mishaps by placing it atop an inverted bowl or other convenient object.

Restaurants

My experiences with restaurants are unlimited, I tell myself as my husband and I prepare to meet three couples for dinner. How can there be any surprises after all these years of meeting good friends at Long Island's vast list of eating places! But of course there are surprises out there, and this night promises to be a memorable experience. The restaurant is famous for brook trout scooped, less than an hour before they appear on dinner plates, from a trout farm in the restaurant's backyard.

It is the socializing in restaurants that is the essential ingredient for my husband and me, not necessarily the exotic food. We meet friends at diners, pizzerias—most anywhere—just to socialize. Home dinner parties take too many hours of preparation stolen from my writing. My friends and I have a slogan, borrowed from the Greyhound Bus Corporation: "Leave the cooking to restaurant chefs." This way we're all happy and relaxed when we get together.

As important as these restaurant get-togethers were in my preimpairment days, they are even more so now. When the field of activities my friends and I could share

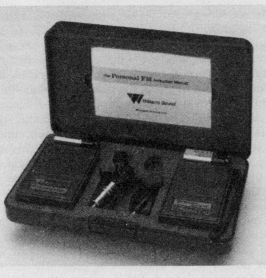

FIGURE 11. The Williams Personal FM System

narrowed (by excluding most movies, theater, opera, concerts, and lectures), restaurants took on enormous social significance.

All restaurants present challenges for people with hearing impairment, but some restaurants are more manageable than others. The normal restaurant noise level becomes impossible when music is piped in. These are restaurants to be avoided by the hearing-impaired unless management is accommodating. Many a time my husband has been able to persuade the manager to save Bruce Springsteen for another time or at least to lower the recording. Some restaurants consider Bruce's blasting voice essential for their clientele (my own children fit this category), a decision I must certainly respect, yet it is a decision I would rather not subject myself to.

This evening we meet friends at a restaurant that

serves Bruce along with brook trout, and while they appreciate my difficulty and place us at a table as far as possible from the speakers piping in Bruce, the fact remains that there is scarcely a piece of territory Bruce's voice does not reach. There is nothing for me to do but make a mental note to check the piped-in music situation in the future before a reservation is made.

This night I will cope as best I can. With the soaring noise, my Williams Sound System has only minimal value. I will have to pass the microphone from one mouth to another. When there are so many seated at the table and various conversations going on at the same time, passing the microphone can be confusing. I need a more creative approach. Because these three couples are such good friends, they join my search for "creative." I do not try for hearing in this restaurant. I have too much hearing: torrents of dialogue; cascading waterfalls of words from our table and the surrounding ones; the clatter of dishes, silverware, and rolling carts; and, of course, Bruce. All this hearing grinds in my ears like a trolley car. What I need is less hearing and a little bit of comprehension.

I turn off my hearing aids and smile at the world around me in welcome relief. My friends say they are also disadvantaged by the noise level, and at times they cup their hands at their ears and frown. Still, when the maitre d' comes to announce the specials, they function well.

I'm always quick to announce my impairment. The obliging maitre d' moves closer. Proximity does not help. This man is so taken with the chef's specials that words roll on his tongue and not a consonant remains in place. My good friend Rose sees the problem. Jumping from her seat, she positions herself at the maitre d's side. Rose is a petite woman with a penchant for taking charge. She will be the interpreter and the maitre d' will assist her by pausing after each sentence.

Rose, my take-charge actress friend, does charades.

Her mouth moves well, and her arms flail about comically as she imitates trout swimming in a farm's fresh water. She demonstrates all the ingenious ways this restaurant features brook trout; the various cooking methods; the cutting, slicing, or halving; the elaborate stuffings.

There is laughter, not only at our table. Rose has made an entertainment for all surrounding tables in this noisy restaurant and is having a significant impact on hearing viewers. There is applause when she inscribes letters in the air. I can sense that others with hearing impairment will profit from her act.

We eight friends make our selections of trout, and on the menu I find a tempting spinach, shiitake mushroom, and walnut salad, which the friend seated next to me also orders. Having made my selections of salad and trout, I relax and try to speechread as far and wide as my eyes can see at this generously oversized oval table.

I glean what I can from various lips moving at dizzying paces, one reply following so fast upon another that my head spins trying to keep all parts of the conversation in sight. Just as I think I am making sense of what is being said, the conversation detours and I am lost. From time to time kind friend Rose, seated opposite me, clues me in or I tug at my husband's sleeve for a hint of the subject that is causing such howls of laughter.

I try, really try, to be part of this world of hearing friends, but my eyes rebel and soon I sit back with my private thoughts. In general, this first part of the evening, the cocktails and bread-nibbling part, is dismal failure. But it is the price of socializing, I tell myself, knowing I would rather be here with my friends than sitting at home the way "dropouts" do. My friend Cynthia tells me she can't tolerate an evening when she doesn't know "what the hell is going on."

I comfort myself that my reward will come with the luscious salad of spinach, mushrooms, and walnuts, and I keep reminding my husband to be sure to remember what is being said so that I will be further rewarded with a pleasant half-hour review of this meal when we get home.

With fanfare a wagon is wheeled to the table, but no salads appear. The waiter does a dance routine, wielding baton-like spoons over and into a caldron of pasta. Someone took the liberty of ordering this appetizer for the whole table, and the salads were canceled with no "lip alert" to me. Problem is, angel hair pasta drenched with tiny wedges of vegetables requires the eyes of the diner to be cast downward. I can observe no lips at the table during this course. The boneless fish is easier. Still, since no fish-boning job is foolproof, my eyes are split between attention to other people's mouths and my own. I do my best. This evening is a nurturing experience—nurturing my patience.

A joke teller three seats away really wants to get a laugh from me. But he has a mouth that remains bunched when he talks; his tongue, teeth, and lips are fused, and his words are shapeless. I read the humor and friendship in his eyes and assure him that my husband will give me the gist and the punch line later.

My friend Rose cannot accept this. She stands to pantomime the story. Her movements are incredibly funny, and our entire table—plus the surrounding ones—are treated to another round of comedy. I do not understand some of the fine nuances, but I love what I have understood and I love my friend Rose for trying so hard to keep me attached to the world of my hearing friends.

Postmortem on the Evening at the Restaurant

"So how was the trout?" Cynthia asks as we take one of our regular walks through our village.

"We'll have to go together sometime."

"I'd like that," Cynthia says. "One of the things I hate

about large groups are the thoughtless indignities. I'm always steeling myself to keep my mouth shut. I mean, I feel like such a fool when I unwittingly interrupt and a supposedly well-meaning friend lets me know someone else has the floor."

"I know the feeling," I tell Cynthia.

"But you're tougher-skinned than I."

"It's just an act," I laugh.

"Makes me so damn mad," Cynthia continues. "It's hard enough for people with hearing impairment to enter group conversations, and the thing is, I'm no interrupter. I mean, in my hearing days I was never an interrupter though interrupting has always been an accepted way of life in social communication. How many times I've been interrupted by a hearing person! No one ever tells the hearing person to wait his or her turn. So why do some hearing people feel compelled to silence me when I interrupt a pair of hidden lips?"

To lighten the mood, I take Cynthia's arm and promise to not interrupt her dissertation on interrupting. We both laugh and Cynthia continues: "For people with a hearing disability to get the thrust of group conversation is a large enough hurdle. Following mouths when there's scarcely a pause from the time one mouth finishes talking to the moment the next mouth begins requires enormous concentration. It's also a feat of athletic agility for our necks and eyes. I mean, when I first became impaired, I'd work so damn hard to understand and not interrupt, but still misunderstandings and interruptions happen.

"I've sat quietly through many a dinner party while mouths at either side of me chewed while talking. I would never correct this way of talking, which happens to be poor manners in addition to making comprehension an impossibility for someone who is hearing impaired. I've stood quietly through animated conversations while hands flailed about, obscuring mouths and pinching and scratching at noses—again, not the finest of manners.

And how about the gum chewing and yawning? I could be a snob and call it crudeness or rudeness, but at best it's an impossibility for people with hearing impairment.

"Still, I kept trying, which means I would sometimes, though infrequently—and always unknowingly—interrupt. I risked embarrassment for misreading or mishearing words or for speaking on a topic that had passed, and I didn't mind corrections by the hearing when I made these mistakes. What I couldn't abide were corrections that would never be given to the hearing. Within the hearing world interruptions are accepted, not corrected. I think people with hearing impairment should get the same tolerance."

"I think those of us with impairment deserve more tolerance," I tell Cynthia, "and I'm sure the hearing friends who silence us when we interrupt mean to be helpful. They can't know that this silencing is a reminder to us of all the other difficulties and indignities we face."

Cynthia is close to tears when she adds, "This kind of silencing scalds us because it's so unfair. When it would happen to me, I had to exert enormous control not to say, 'Why don't you silence your hearing pals when *they* interrupt?' It's as though the hearing make a separate society for us, putting us in the category of children. Well, damn it, it's only our ears that are faulty. No one has to take me by the arm and say, 'Cynthia, so-and-so is talking.' "

I tell Cynthia, "Just as we must put up with other indignities to remain part of the hearing world, so do we have to tough it out within group conversations. We must hope that greater awareness of our problem will bring greater sensitivity. What we all need are more friends like my friend Rose and more friends like my friend Fran (with a Boston accent that causes me no end of difficulty), who will stand on her head, if need be, until I understand her New England English.

"But I appreciate what you're saying about interrupting. I've had that upsetting experience too often myself.

It's slowed me down when I'm in groups, but I refuse to let it make me stop participating. Sometimes I'll ask a member of the group, 'Is anyone else speaking now?' I've even announced in groups that I want to participate but don't want to interrupt and that if they all keep their mouths visible to me, I'll have a better chance of seeing what's being said and I'll be able to participate more intelligently.

"Good friends assure me they don't object if I unwittingly interrupt. I've gone on a campaign about this within my circle of friends. What it comes down to is this: How eager are your hearing friends to have you as part of their group! How much do they appreciate your friendship!

"Friends and family of the hearing-impaired have to find new ways to relate to us once we are impaired. And we must also work at finding new ways to relate to our hearing friends and family. In a sense, we learn new appreciation of friends and family. I think this working together makes both us and the hearing stronger and more valuable to ourselves and to others."

The R section of my Rolodex bulges with restaurants I have rated not only for excellence of food but for excellence of acoustics. From Long Island's milelong list, I have singled out my favorites, always keeping in mind that on a Saturday night any restaurant can fail the noise-level test. Another feature, besides the piped-in music, that places restaurants on a hearing-impaired person's rejection list is the decor factor. A restaurant with cushioned seats, curtained windows, and carpeting has the best environment for impaired ears.

There is a nervous energy in crowded restaurants that translates to raucous interference when it comes to hearing aids. I can avoid some of this crowd stress in diners and pizzerias by eating in a booth. When no booth is available, I look for a corner space and choose the seat furthest from other tables. My Williams Sound System is sometimes an effective aid. When I tell the waiter I am hearing impaired, a frequent response is "Oh, I'm sorry," a response I always feel deserves reassurance. I tell the waiter that I'll manage well with his cooperation, and hold the microphone of my Williams Sound System close to his mouth. The outcome is usually satisfactory.

No restaurant experience is excellent for the hearing-impaired; it is a matter of selecting the least difficult situation. Ideally, there should be only one couple with my husband and me. Seated alongside a friend, I can understand most of what he or she says, and assistive aids are unnecessary. Since my eyes will be diverted to my friend's lips, I must make careful choices of food. What I eat is of secondary importance; my primary concern is to understand the conversation.

For serious eating, my husband and I can go to restaurants without friends. People with hearing impairment must make choices when handling the restaurant challenge.

A Garden Wedding

Through the lovely ritual of a garden wedding I am disconnected. Eyeing the bride and groom, the minister, and the attendants in pastels that upstage the beds of summer flowers, I hear nothing. I had prepared myself for not hearing, yet it is disconcerting when it happens. Controlling disappointment, I open myself to the beauty of what could be a silent film; I am just part of a crowd for whom the talkies have not yet dawned. I guess this is as good a way of viewing the scene as any, and at least I am among good friends who later will share with me the minister's words and the very special vows the bride and groom have written for themselves.

In faces around me I can see the vows are very touch-

ing. This is a wedding I have particularly been looking
forward to. The bride is the daughter of a very dear college friend, who until recently has been moaning that she
will never have the joy of seeing her daughter enter a
traditional union.

The wedding is almost traditional except for the personal vows, which, my friend has alerted me, are more
preachy than vows, and the decor, which is not berib-
boned and flower-decked, other than nature's natural
bloom.

The scene could be Walden Pond's park, with rustic
tables and everything biodegradable, including the
groom's paper carnation. One of the caveats to the mother
of the bride declared the cutting of flowers a travesty and
a rudeness to nature. There is enough for my eyes to take
in, although for this first part of the afternoon I may as
well have left my ears at home.

Dance music, which takes over when the minister is
done, is a string quartet backed up by a guitar duet. The
dance floor, nature's green carpet, fills with young people
who find a way to move with the rhythm of Joan Baez and
Pete Seeger specialties. We in the generation at the far end
of the gap blend gradually with the young dancers.

I try to minimize anxiety whenever I'm invited to dance
by offering an explanation of my problem; still, my hearing partner, so schooled in talking while dancing, usually
reverts to his original habit and I am lost. This happens
when the father of the bride invites me for a spin on the
grass. The afternoon takes a pleasant turn when I begin
to mix with the younger set.

I've always enjoyed the company of my children's
friends and am quite at home when the bride makes me a
celebrity among her peers. Everyone wants to know about
the book I am writing, and invitations to dance are plenti-
ful from the groom and his good men. There is much I
learn about these young people. They are quick to understand my difficulty, and they absorb my impairment with

grace, passing information from one to another within their group. They all exhibit skill and sensitivity. Mouths turn to face me, and I become a full partner in their afternoon of banter. Again and again I am invited to dance, and their dancing is as splendid as their chatter. No hefty embraces keep my eyes looking over shoulders where I can see no lip movement. Instead, I am kept at arm's length so my eyes can retain contact with mouths opposite me. My partners and I do individual body movements, but our eyes and mouths are in close touch.

I am treated to the manual alphabet, in which many of these young people are proficient. And they are generous with body language. Perhaps the gap between us makes these young people less self-conscious about working with my impairment. It may just be that for many of my contemporaries I am a frightening example of what the aging process may have in store for them so they unwittingly set themselves apart from my impairment by not really trying to work with it.

At any rate, this afternoon is a tremendous success, and I regret the sunset that ends the Saturday wedding celebration. The largest challenge this day has been taking leave of my own generation to embrace these loving, caring, understanding young people.

Bridge Nuts

Reaching for new ways to socialize, I investigate opportunities. Bridge is both old and new for me. In preimpairment days my friends Helen and Charlie became bridge addicted. When Charlie retired from dentistry, bridge became his life.

Charlie, who was earning master points and teaching and playing bridge seven nights a week, had trouble pulling me into his obsession. My husband and I remained "sometimes" or "once in a while" bridge players. Then there were my neighbors Jules and Lil. A bridge aficionado but not the addict Charlie was, Jules invited my husband and me to join his two-table monthly bridge evening.

Hearing impairment had begun limiting many of the ways my husband and I could socialize so, as a social statement I think, we embraced the card game.

My friend Cynthia asked, "What do you find so engrossing about bridge?"

"Its most engrossing feature is that it's something people with hearing impairment *can do.*"

"You think we have to invent ways to socialize?" Her voice was stern, teacherlike, even a bit aggressive, I thought, and when I answered my voice also had a teacherlike stern edge: "I think we had better."

"Why should people with hearing impairment play bridge if it doesn't appeal to them?"

"It doesn't have to be bridge," I tell Cynthia. "Other card games would be fine also. I just happen to think bridge is an intelligent and thoughtful game, a game of constant challenge. Since we are no strangers to challenge, bridge is, I think, ideally suited to us."

"So how does one learn the game?"

I answered in Cynthia's flat tone: "One registers for a bridge class."

Reluctantly, Cynthia agreed to give it a try. Long Island is fertile territory for new and old bridge players. A young woman called Roberta 'sez' so ("Roberta Sez" is her logo). Roberta says bridge can be learned in a class of two hundred (50 bridge tables) where she bellows instructions, interlaced with her special brand of humor, into a microphone. Cynthia enrolled. However, she understood not one word and didn't return for lesson number two.

"My husband and I will help you with basics," I offered. Cynthia, her husband, my husband, and I became a foursome at her kitchen table or at mine. Cynthia is a bright woman and caught on quickly. But catching on to basics does not a bridge player make. What else could I do for Cynthia? I investigated Roberta and her class of two hundred. I could only understand what Roberta had to say by reading her instruction sheets. When she taught the fine points, sang, joked, and rocked and rolled with her portable microphone, I was lost. I called on my Williams Sound System. Roberta was generous enough to work with the Williams System. She attached the lapel-clip microphone and kept the transmitter in her jacket pocket. I heard with such amazing clarity that I had to remind myself that I am hearing impaired.

This experience was similar to my experience with the loop at a SHHH meeting. These assistive aids can turn a life around, and I wish I could broadcast this good news to my hearing-impaired comrades everywhere.

Cynthia gave Roberta "Sez" a second chance, and her purchase of a Williams Sound System was the beginning of socializing. My dropout friend is a new woman. For the first time she talks with enthusiasm about the forthcoming bar mitzvah for her twin sons. The past months had been filled with gloom as she bemoaned the fact that she, the mother of these wonderful boys, would not know the joy of hearing them talk and sing on this grand occasion.

The experience of understanding every word Roberta had to say to a class of two hundred gave zest to Cynthia's days. She talks about finding a new career. I know that bridge teacher Roberta inspired her, but larger credit goes to the Williams Sound System for giving her the ability to be in communication with a part of the hearing world from which she had been isolated.

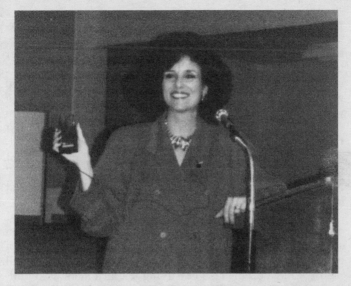

FIGURE 12. A bridge teacher with the Williams FM Transmitter (Photo by Phil Mayer)

The Hearing-Impaired Mother of Bar Mitzvah Twins

It was an affair of many double joys. Daniel and Josh, Cynthia's twin sons, spoke and sang to Cynthia's impaired ears and mine. Two microphone buttons and two transmitters from two Williams Sound Systems sat on the lectern. Josh tested the instruments before the service began, asking his mother and me if we could hear him.

When Cynthia raised her hand to acknowledge that she was tuned in to her sons, I saw a very different young woman from the one I had met several months before. She was no longer the dropout. The proud young voice of her son Daniel reached the assembled family and friends: "We want our mother and her good friend to hear us, so we're going to speak very carefully." Tears in many eyes acknowledged these special children who were unashamed of their mother's predicament and were eager to make her a part of their hearing world.

I was reminded of my own granddaughter Rebecca, who moves her mouth so well for me that I never miss a word she says no matter the din within the room, out in the street, or in the yard. One day I took Rebecca, just turned eight, to our village pool. Rebecca stood up to address the women I was sitting with: "You don't talk right to my grandmother. I can show you how to speak to her." My granddaughter gave a lesson in mouth movement that has become a classic in our small village.

Cynthia's twins and Rebecca exemplify what is best and so admirable about children. They learn quickly and stand ready to help tune in the hearing world for those of us with hearing loss. Some hearing-impaired friends tell me they have other, less gratifying, experiences with children. I suggest they try harder. I truly believe that children like Josh, Daniel, and Rebecca, little people in a complicated universe, can change the hearing world for people with impairment.

Dear friend the Williams Sound System also reunites the impaired with the hearing world. The small button microphone and transmitter make it possible for people with hearing impairment to enjoy lectures, religious services, political forums, small or large reading groups, guided museum tours, large groups of people at social gatherings, and small groups of friends in a home. All that is required is a willing lecturer or friend, like bridge teacher Roberta, to use the Williams equipment and people with hearing impairment to introduce the hearing to the special equipment that can connect the two worlds.*

---

* FM hearing aids described by Steven Malawer, Audiologist, on page 229 offer a hearing system similar to the Williams Sound System.

Chapter 7

Medicine Men

Hospitals and Doctors

This gloomy afternoon, as I learn to manage a broken wrist, Cynthia and I switch roles. I am the dropout, sullen as I complain about emergency facilities at our community hospital and incensed that people with hearing impairment are second-class citizens.

I had slipped the previous evening and broken the fall with my right hand. The young doctor who attended me in the emergency room of our community hospital (one of Long Island's finest) spoke in a fast, wiry voice more suited to the floor of the commodities exchange than a treatment room for people in pain.

"I'd like to understand what you're saying," I told him as he examined my X-rays and mumbled various options I might consider. His mumbling continued and when I interrupted, insisting he accommodate my hearing impairment, he returned to his fast-paced, wiry speech. There were probably few other physicians available, since it was close to midnight, or I'd have asked for another doctor to take over.

After I instructed the young physician in the proper way to talk to a person with hearing impairment, he spoke only to my husband. It was as though I'd evaporated. I was severed from my wrist, which became a property to be tossed between the doctor and my husband.

I had two options, my husband told me, translating for me as though I were a child—a hard or soft cast. I felt myself choking beneath a blanket of tears. I had many questions that needed answers: Which type of cast would make it easier for a writer in the midst of a project to function with? Which type of cast was better for the wrist? How long would the healing take? Would there be lasting damage? I could have used my husband as a conduit, directing questions to the doctor through him, but something in me rebelled. I guess the pain did it. Or maybe the years of holding back when hearing people lacked proper consideration. Or maybe I was just terribly tired and low-spirited. I told my husband he could drive me home and in the morning I'd go to a hand doctor I had heard about.

The young emergency room physician was a doctor in need of doctoring. He should have learned in medical school that healing is a total process. He should have known that even a child patient deserves to be brought into the decision-making process to help determine which treatment will best promote healing. For this young man to ignore me and deal exclusively with my husband was not only an insult, it was a warning that his doctoring might be as faulty as his knowledge about accommodating hearing-impaired patients. Better to suffer out the night and go to a proper doctor in the morning.

I cradled my broken wrist in my other hand as though I were smuggling it out of that nasty place. Walking through the emergency section of the hospital, I felt strangely embarrassed that I had permitted myself to slip and break a piece of me. Half-blinded by pain, I wished I were one of the other people rushing past me. Anyone else—orderly, nurse, person mopping the floor. Anyone with hearing ears. How could I have been careless enough, I demanded of myself, to slip at the time of night when one must depend upon the emergency room at a hospital! How could I have been careless enough to slip at all! Bad enough having broken ears; why break another part of me! Home at last, my body was a block of ice during a July heat spell. My husband kept covering me with blankets, all the while regretting that I hadn't allowed the emergency room doctor to relieve my pain with a cast.

I was consumed with regrets of my own. The night was endless with pain and regret. I screamed inwardly that I must stop picking on myself, but I tearfully continued, teeth chattering, until it was morning.

The hand doctor was an example of what doctors should be. He spoke carefully and directly to me. When I didn't understand a word, he wrote notes for me. His kindness, understanding, and willingness to work with my impairment should have healed my broken spirits, but the hospital emergency room trauma remained with me.

Walking with Cynthia, I feel very much the dropout she had been. "We people with hearing impairment got one bum deal," I say.

"Hey, think positive," Cynthia answers. "You could have broken a leg."

"Don't humor me," I tell her.

"Think about the very good doctor. And think about the article you can write offering hints to young doctors who need to learn there's more to healing bones than casts. Doctors need to know that the spirit of a hearing-impaired person can be broken more easily than a bone and that the healing can be far more complicated."

My friend Cynthia helped me put the hospital emergency room experience in perspective. She helped me establish rules for myself if ever I should find myself in a hospital again. And she helped me consider practical guides for the hearing-impaired in a hospital.

A Guide for the Hearing-Impaired Hospitalized Patient

People with hearing impairment are disadvantaged in any large institution or facility. Because a hospital experience for people with hearing impairment can be traumatic, it is most advisable that they have a member of the family or a close friend see them through the experience.

Doctors should be acquainted with the patient's history of hearing impairment and should have thorough knowledge of ototoxic medicines. Ideally, doctors, nurses, and other hospital personnel would be educated by the hospital in how to talk to the hearing-impaired, but family and friends can also help educate doctors and nurses in how to deal with patients who are hearing disabled.

The hospital room of a hearing-impaired person should have a large, legible sign on the door explaining that the patient is hearing impaired. Similar signs should hang from the front of the bed and be taped above it. These signs must be conspicuous so that every nurse, orderly, doctor, and administrator in any capacity is immediately alerted that the patient is hearing impaired. It can be terrifying for the hearing-impaired patient to be aroused or intruded upon for a procedure when the person doing the rousing or intruding is not aware that the patient is hearing disabled.

Nurses, doctors, and others entering the room of a hearing-impaired person should first determine if the patient is wearing hearing aids—or has removed them and therefore needs to locate and insert them in order to understand what is about to be done to his or her body. Medical personnel should be equipped with pencil and paper so that, if necessary, a message can be written to the patient. Having a friend or family member monitor what happens in the room of a hearing-impaired patient is advisable, particularly when the patient comes from surgery.

A Model Program

Chicago's Michael Reese Humana Hospital has a model program for the hearing-impaired, deaf, or blind patient. Carol Beckenstein, who directs this volunteer program, explained it to me: "The program was developed in 1988. It is color coded—red for low vision, green for hearing impairment. The coding provides nonverbal communication between staff and patient. Staff immediately knows the patient has a disability. For the hearing-impaired we have amplifier phones, television decoders, headphones, signers, interpreters, and pocketalkers. And if a patient requests an assistive device we don't have, we can usually provide it promptly.

"Patients were originally evaluated by admitting personnel who were very rushed and not trained to pick up disabilities like hearing impairment. Now volunteers in the patient relations program, who have special training, do the evaluating. Volunteers visit patients and are trained to pick up disabilities so that patients can be included in the program. I must emphasize, this program is not only for the elderly. The first patient in the pilot program was a very young deaf woman who had given birth.

"There are of course the difficulties of personnel changes, so the training of doctors, nurses, and orderlies is ongoing. We would like to see our program adopted by other hospitals. Northwestern University Hospital is now using the program in a slightly different format."

Ruth Green and Sue Bromberg, co-coordinators of *advocates for better communication* (a.b.c.), a volunteer group allied with the League for the Hard of Hearing, organized two kits that belong in every health care facility and every home library of every person with a hearing loss.

The first kit, *Hearing Health Care Program for Medical Facilities,* assists a facility to meet the needs of the hospitalized person with a hearing difficulty. It includes information on how to set up a program to train hospital staff and comes complete with identification stickers, a page of suggested ways to communicate with someone who has a hearing loss, a glossary of terms with which the facility personnel should be familiar, information about securing interpreter services, and a list of assistive devices it is suggested the facility should make available. The kit contains order forms for a videotape demonstrating the care of patients with hearing loss and an audiotape to provide sensitivity training for staff. Patients with hearing problems will be well served by the medical facility that has this kit. For information or to order, call 212-741-3143, or fax 212-255-4413.

The second kit, *For Consumers with a Hearing Loss: A Kit for Better Health Access,* should be in the home of every person with a hearing loss. It is the number one item to be put in a travel bag that is being prepared for a hospital experience. This a.b.c. kit tells people with hearing loss that they need to take responsibility for their care and explains how to do so when they are to be hospitalized. This kit will help the patient know his or her entitlements and just how to go about taking much of the pain out of a hospital stay. There are also sample letters to be followed if the patient did not receive entitlements. The kit includes all this and more for a nominal charge of $3. To order or for more information, call 212-255-1932 (TTY) or 212-741-3143 (voice).

The Implant

During our long walks Cynthia and I talk past fractured bones and hospital etiquette to recent scientific advances with great promise for the hearing-impaired. When I visited the House Ear Institute in California in 1985, the implant they were using gave the profoundly impaired the ability to recognize environmental sounds. A young woman I interviewed explained why she braved the operation, which was then in its infancy.

Connie Martinez-Wild Tells Her Story

"My hearing disability is hereditary. It is a progressive loss. Two of my sons have early hearing problems. I began using a hearing aid when I was about eight years old. As I grew older I had more and more difficulty understanding what was being said. The loss in both my ears became profound, yet I could use a hearing aid in one ear. This is most unusual. No one knows why. My disability made me very shy and introverted.

"As a single parent, I became frightened about the idea of not being able to use even the one hearing aid. This could happen. And if it did, how would I be able to manage as a single parent and provide for my family? I decided to look into the implant for the ear that couldn't use a hearing aid. The implant would be a backup for me if I was no longer able to use the aid. I also had another reason for wanting to have the implant: I would be helping with research that might someday benefit my children.

"The implant has given me a lot of confidence. With it I can pick up sound on both sides. I'm not so fearful anymore. I've become outgoing. The internal implant coil by itself doesn't help me hear. I have an external device that acts like a hearing aid. This external device, the size of a pack of cigarettes, is much smaller and easier to wear than the first one I had. The implant has greatly improved my life. It has helped me acknowledge my disability. With the implant in one ear and an aid in the other ear, I manage very well.

"I work for the House Ear Institute. I work with children after they have the implant. With the audiologist, I help train the child to use the new sounds heard with the implant."

Connie now works at the Catholic Charities of Orange County. She recently wrote to me saying, "The cochlear implant has been instrumental in helping me discover myself and my capabilities. Because of the implant and my many years with the House Ear Institute, I am in a position to better understand deafness and its implications. Today I work for Catholic Charities, coordinating the Deaf Outreach Services program. The experiences, knowledge, and skills I gained in the past ten years opened new doors that allow me to serve deaf and hearing-impaired people and their families. I've come a long way, and I'm proud of the accomplishments which I have and continue to experience. I owe Dr. Bill House and the House Ear Institute a world of thanks."

Connie Martinez-Wild was a pioneer. The current implant is a remarkable advance.

My Friend Charlotte Roth Explains Her Implant

"I will start with the background of my hearing loss. I started to lose my hearing in my late thirties and early forties. First the loss was in one ear. Then I started to lose my hearing in my second ear. The loss was mild to moderate for many, many years. About five years ago my hearing loss began to increase rather rapidly, and over a period of several months my hearing loss went from moderate to severe in both ears.

"With the assistance of my 'telephone switch' hearing aids, I was able to function. But as time went on, even those became useless to me. My severely impaired hearing deteriorated to the profound level. I now had to rely on speechreading almost one hundred percent. My hearing impairment, which began as mild and finally became profound, happened over a period of about twenty years.

"With profound impairment, it was almost impossible for me to function on a day-to-day basis in my work and in my social life. I found it extremely difficult to manage. I became a candidate for the *cochlear implant* when the protocol was changed.

"On April 11, 1990, I was operated on at the Manhattan Eye, Ear, and Throat Hospital. I was hooked up by May 15, 1990. The initial sounds I heard were both wonderful and awful. There were sounds I had not heard in maybe ten years. However, the clarity of the sounds was very different from anything I could remember hearing in the past. Everything sounded scratchy or squeaky. Sounds were a little like comic strip characters. Like animated cartoons. Like artificially synthesized speech.

"It was very difficult for me to make anything out of the sounds I initially heard. But over a period of time I began to be able to identify various environmental sounds from my past: my cats, the doorbell, the telephone ringing, car horns. Those sounds became very easy for me to identify. Then I found it was very easy to speechread because the sounds I was hearing began to make sense. I was beginning to be able to understand without needing to watch the speaker's face every single minute.

"After a while I was even able to understand sounds on the radio, and I reached the point where I could understand the complete weather report on the radio. The vocabulary in a weather report is pretty predictable, so that wasn't very difficult. I could also hear almost the entire stock report on the radio. Numbers came across very clearly; they did very early on after my cochlear implant.

"During the news section of a radio program, I can understand between forty and fifty percent of what is being said. I cannot understand all the fine points, but I can identify the topic that is being discussed. Combining my knowledge of the subject, I can generally get a good idea of what is being talked about.

"There are three hospitals within the metropolitan area that do the cochlear implant: Manhattan Eye, Ear, and Throat Hospital, New York University Hospital, and Einstein Medical Center.

"You really need to do a lot of research on your own to make the decision about which hospital to go to for the surgery. Also about which doctor to choose. Some otolaryngologists and audiologists may be able to direct you or make recommendations. In my case, no one directed me. I had to seek out the information myself. I read every article I could find on the subject.

"I had been reading about the cochlear implant for six or seven years, going back to the time it was only a single channel implant. When the *Nucleus 22-Channel Cochlear Implant System* was first introduced, I went for an evaluation to see if I would be eligible. But at that very early stage, doctors did not perform the surgery on people who fell into the severely impaired category. They were not permitted to. The candidate had to be profoundly impaired. I was rejected but I kept discussing my eagerness for the implant with my otolaryngologist.

"When the FDA widened its scope for candidates for the cochlear implant, my otolaryngologist contacted me. He explained that with my hearing loss I was now a candidate for the cochlear implant. I then made contacts and arranged for an evaluation.

"I'm not a physician but I can describe the procedure based on my personal knowledge and experience. Basically, what you have with the implant is an internal mechanism and an external part of the implant.

"Internally, the device is implanted through the mastoid bone of one ear. The implant consists of a magnet and a receiver and twenty-two electrodes. The electrodes are wired into the cochlea. They are snaked into that little snail-shaped component of the inner ear. The magnet is placed right under the scalp and right next to the electronic receiver.

"Externally, you wear another device that is a transmitter which has a magnet in the center of it. A small wire attaches this to a microphone which looks very much like a behind-the-ear hearing aid. It sits over your ear like a behind-the-ear hearing aid except that you don't need ear molds in your ear if it stays on properly. If it does not fit securely, you may have to use molds in the ear to keep it in place.

"The transmitter, which is a circular device about an inch and a half in diameter, has a wire that connects both the microphone wire and the transmitter wire. They are joined into one wire which goes down and goes into a small boxlike device about the size of a pack of cigarettes. This is the speech processor. Actually, it is a small computer.

"The sounds in the environment are picked up by the microphone that sits behind your ear. This sound travels through the microphone, down the short wire, into the long wire, into the speech processor.

"The speech processor has been programmed by an audiologist to select and filter sound that is appropriate for you, specifically for you, to enable you to understand speech. These sounds then go back up the wire into the transmitter, which is sitting on the side of your head. The transmitter transmits this sound across your scalp to the receiver, which is sitting just under it.

"The receiver takes this electronic message and sends it through the twenty-two wires that have been inserted into your cochlea; the electronic signal is then sent to the auditory nerve; and the brain repeats the message of sound, which you then interpret as something in your environment—a person talking, a dog barking, a telephone ringing.

"One of the many wonders of my cochlear implant has been my ability to use the telephone. I was very fortunate. I was able to begin using the telephone three months after surgery. The equipment I use on my telephone is actually designed to assist when you are tape-recording a telephone conversation. It is designed to be plugged into a tape recorder and a telephone. The one I use is a Radio Shack adaptor, which works very well with my implant device. It works with the speech processor, the cigarette-pack-like box I wear, which has an input; I plug this device right into the input space that connects directly to the telephone line, so I get a much clearer sound and I eliminate some of the distortion that occurs through the handset amplifier.

"There is another adaptor that is more portable, also available at Radio Shack. It is a little suction cup device that is placed on the receiver of the telephone. The other end is plugged into the speech processor. I've used this device less successfully. Sometimes it works, sometimes it doesn't. It depends on the connection you have on the phone and quality of the voice of the speaker at the other end.

"In general, my ability, since the implant, to use the telephone is miraculous.

"Unfortunately, several months ago I had an incident of Ménière's syndrome. It affected my inner ear, which in turn affected the sounds I was getting from my processor.

"What happened between then and now is that we have tried about fifteen to twenty different programs to get the sound back to where it was, and so far we have made small inroads but have not been successful in getting it all the way back.

"Part of the process is probably going to be my healing from Ménière's syndrome, which happened to be totally unrelated to the implant. Ménière's syndrome is a problem I had several times in my life prior to the implant.

"The cost of a cochlear implant is twenty-six or twenty-seven thousand dollars. Most insurance companies cover the cost of the Nucleus 22-Channel Cochlear Implant because it is approved by the FDA. My insurance company paid for almost everything. I only had to pay a little more than a thousand dollars out of pocket.

"The programming after the implant surgery is included in the cost, up to a certain point. I am not sure where that point is. I have had well over a hundred different 'maps,' and I am now on a complete program. There are different programs used for different implant patients. There is a specific program for people in the profound range and a specific program for people in the severe range.

"I had been using the program for people in the severe range. It worked very very well for me until I had the problem with Ménière's syndrome. But when we could not get that program back to where it was, the audiologist, in consultation with the cochlear specialist, decided to switch my program entirely to see if I could do better with the profound protocol. I am on that program now.

"Between the two programs, I have had well over a hundred 'maps.' A map is a schedule of sounds that is put into your computer every time you go for an adjustment. Each time you go for an adjustment, you try three, four, or five different maps. When I say I've been through well over a hundred maps, I don't mean I've gone to be programmed a hundred times.

"During a session you try some map, and you know instantly it is no good. Then you try something else, and you know instantly that it is good. So in any one session you may go through five or ten maps, depending upon what the problem is.

"Most people do not sleep with the external units of the implant. They clip right off. The unit is about an inch behind your ear just about where the mastoid bone is located. That's where the surgery is performed, right through the mastoid bone.

"Most people unclip the unit when they go to sleep. I did initially. I wore it fourteen to fifteen hours a day in the beginning. Now, I rarely remove it. I sleep with it. I take it off when I shower, of course. I also remove the unit when I'm doing some work in the house I think might damage the mechanism. Otherwise, I wear it twenty-two to twenty-three hours a day, most every day of the week.

"There is a long process that you have to go through before you are accepted as a candidate for the transplant. The degree of your hearing loss is only the first step to see if you are within the FDA allowable limit. Once that is determined, you have interviews with an audiologist, your surgeons, a speech therapist. I had evaluations for almost two months. A candidate's motivation is crucial.

"There is a great deal of hard work to be done by the implant patient. High motivation is a most important factor in determining who will be a candidate for the implant."

Chapter 8

Entertainment

Joy and Challenge

Entertainment cannot be taken for granted by people with hearing impairment. Old pleasures, like old habits, need to be changed.

There is no simple selecting from available movies when a free evening comes up; no flipping of the channel selector to choose whichever TV program seems tempting; no ordering of theater tickets when a new show is reviewed or standing in a twofer line, ready to grab most any tempting bargain. Every entertainment needs careful planning.

Television

When hearing impairment is mild, it is often the hearing members of the family, not the impaired one, who are disadvantaged. The impaired are not being selfish when they turn the TV volume high; they think their volume setting is in the normal range. Only when complaints are made do they realize how annoying the accommodation to their need can be to the normal ear.

When my impairment was mild, my husband and I watched very little television; when we did, we frequently watched on separate sets several rooms apart. When my impairment became moderate, the volume I required caused distortion. I learned to use an assistive aid that buttoned onto my hearing aid. To use this device, a television set must have a headphone jack (not all sets do). The button-on device has a cord that hooks into the headphone jack on the TV set. Connected directly into the TV set, I was able to enjoy most programs. Those that gave me trouble featured dubbed-in voices, British accents, fast-paced speech, and excessive background music.

Not all hearing aids are equipped with this button-on TV attachment. When I needed a new hearing aid, the replacement did not have the TV device. My audiologist helped me develop my own personal listening system: an ear mold attached by an earphone cable that hooked into the TV headphone jack. This system worked well until my impairment became severe; my discrimination deteriorated and my personal listening system was no longer effective.

My husband and I were deprived of our nightly hour of relaxing with the TV, which was housed in a unit in front of our bed. No longer could we watch Public Broadcasting's appealing shows (or even something mindless that would act as a soporific). Then a friend told me about captioning. Closed captioning returned a flow of entertainment to our household.

Every morning now, no matter how vital the news on page one, it is the television page I turn to first. I am not a television addict. In fact, I have little acquaintance with most of the popular shows. This poring over television offerings every morning, even before I glance at the weather prediction, is neither an idle compulsion nor a psychological quirk. Nothing is wrong with my head except the ears at either side of it.

As is true for others in the hearing-impaired community, my only visual news source, and my only opportunity to see English-speaking movies or documentaries, is closed-captioned television. Closed-captioned means that subtitles will appear on the TV screen that is connected to a TeleCaption decoder.

Since not all programs are captioned, I search and select among those with the double-*C* logo (CC) or the registered trademark (🖳) of the National Captioning Institute (NCI) for opportunities to tape for my library of videocassettes.

The National Captioning Institute, a nonprofit corporation, was established in 1979 with federal seed funds. When I interviewed John Ball, president of the National Captioning Institute, he explained that the concept of captioning was demonstrated in 1971 in Knoxville, Tennessee, at a National Deaf Educators Conference. National Captioning Institute has its main headquarters in Falls Church, Virginia, and has additional facilities in Hollywood, California, and New York City. There are others who do captioning, but NCI is the sole manufacturer and distributor of TeleCaption decoders. Closed captioning does not mean that subtitles automatically appear on sets wired into decoders; members of the family who wish to view without subtitles simply do not activate the decoder.

Subtitles can only be activated if the program has been captioned. In 1980 NCI offered 16 hours a week of captioned programs. By 1991 NCI offered more than four hundred hours of captioned programs weekly. In 1991 the Department of Education appropriated more than five million dollars to help fund captioning of national newscasts, sports, movies, syndicated programs, and children's programs. The networks, program producers, cable TV suppliers, home video companies, syndicators, and advertisers also contract with NCI to caption programs.

Federal funding and the support of the television in-

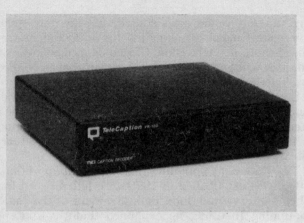

FIGURE 13. A TeleCaption decoder

dustry have enabled the severely impaired and the deaf to enjoy the evening news, prime-time programs on major networks, sports events, cable and syndicated shows, and thousands of home videos. For a small investment (miniscule when compared to the cost of producing a program) severely impaired and deaf people have been able to participate in the hearing world's television. The cost of captioning a half hour of news is under one thousand dollars.

In October 1990 the president signed into law (effective July 3, 1993) a requirement that all new television sets with 13-inch or larger screens have built-in decoder circuitry. This built-in chip would make captioning available to the many families who need but cannot afford a second unit in order to view television. It is estimated that 80 percent of the families who would profit from captioning do not have TeleCaption decoders.

Captioning can advantage a large segment of the hearing population. Studies show that children's reading skills are greatly improved by watching programs with captions. While Nintendo promises to bring forth a computer-skilled generation, captioning can bring forth a generation of readers. Captions are also an excellent tool for people learning English as a second language.

My hearing friend Helen tells me captioning has improved her relations with her hearing-impaired husband. She used to be unable to control her annoyance with the volume he required. And my hearing friend Sally says she is grateful for captioning. She and her hearing husband no longer feel guilty that their deaf child is shut out. All three watch captioned programs together.

It is probably the dream of all who are hearing impaired or deaf that one day soon all television programs will be captioned. It is also our dream that captioning will overcome some of its snags. At times captioned programs have poor contrast and subtitles can scarcely be read. At times phrases or whole paragraphs are omitted. Sometimes captions appear so briefly that dialogue cannot be read by an average reader. In fairness to those who give us captioning, it should be noted that captions are adversely affected by poor reception and other transmission problems.

At times TV listings will omit the double-*C* symbol or the NCI trademark indicating closed captioning when the program in fact is captioned. At other times newspaper listings will erroneously show these symbols next to a program the hearing-impaired and deaf are so eager to see that they alter their other plans; it is with extreme disappointment that they then discover that the program is not captioned.

In the advertising and production of captioned programs there are many imperfections. True, even in the hearing world all is not perfect, though in the world of hearing impairment there is considerably less perfection. But despite these imperfections, those of us who are impaired or deaf are profoundly grateful for captioning.

Movies

When hearing impairment is mild, most English-speaking films can still be enjoyed. When actors have thick British accents, there may be difficult moments, and movie theaters with poor acoustics may create problems. But the mildly impaired person wearing good hearing aids will generally have the same access to movies the hearing community has.

When impairment becomes moderate to severe, find out which movie theaters offer special systems. Many movie theaters are equipped with assistive listening devices to benefit people with hearing impairment. Frequently, there is a notice at the ticket seller's booth about such devices. A phone call to a movie theater to inquire about their equipment for people with hearing difficulty can also be helpful. If the theater has no equipment for people with hearing impairment, there should be a pleasant reminder about the Americans with Disabilities Act. Movie theater managers are usually responsive.

People with hearing disabilities who have been unable to enjoy popular English-speaking films in the theater can take heart. Now most of these films are available on tape, and many are captioned. With a small rental fee and the patience to wait for a current hit to be available on tape, the hearing handicapped can join the hearing world of movie enjoyment. And, of course, foreign films with subtitles enable people with hearing impairment to sit alongside the hearing in movie theaters. Here we are all equal—an emotionally satisfying experience.

My friend Fran, always solicitous of my impairment, has given me a gift subscription to *New York* magazine so that I can store its movie guide for the year. The previous year's new films are frequently captioned on videotapes. In addition, I subscribe to *Silent News*, "the world's most popular newspaper for the deaf" (see Publications for the

Hearing-Impaired in the Directory of Resources at the back of the book). *Silent News* has video reviews of movies that are captioned.

Theater

The mildly and moderately impaired can enjoy productions in theaters using infrared listening systems installed by Sound Associates. Special headphones are available at theaters throughout the country. For the moderately and severely impaired, Sound Associates in New York City offers a neck "loop," which must be arranged for in advance. Telephone 212-586-4167, and a loop will be at the theater for the performance you plan to attend.

The Theater Access Project of Theater Development Fund (TDF) offers low-priced admission tickets for certain Broadway and off-Broadway plays. TDF tries to accommodate patrons with physical or hearing impairment by offering suitable seat locations. To be on the mailing list write or telephone 1501 Broadway, New York, NY 10036, 212-221-0013.

Most live theater houses have infrared or other listening systems. Many houses of worship and other centers also have listening systems. For the severely to profoundly impaired ear that cannot make use of listening systems in New York's Broadway theaters, there is an alternative. The Lincoln Center Library has a special room where scripts for new Broadway productions can be read.

I have communicated with people in the deaf community who attend theater with their hearing mates. They read the script, as I do, beforehand and then, knowing what is happening, thoroughly enjoy the visual experience. These members of the deaf community do not let their differentness interfere with their participation in their hearing mate's entertainment pleasures.

Chapter 9

Ears and Careers

The year my impairment went downhill, from moderate to severe, I grappled with the fact that impaired hearing could end many pleasant events in my average routine. The world as I knew it was pulling away from me. Voices were receding, and I reached out fruitlessly to understand what was being said.

Perhaps the hearing can get an inkling of the feeling if desperation for sound is translated to desperation for food: remember newspaper photographs of Kurdish refugees or victims of the Bangladesh cyclone or the Somalia famine desperately reaching for packages of food. Now visualize the food packages, almost within reach of outstretched arms, receding, unattainable; each time the arm extends to grab a morsel, the food recedes still further. This is how it is when the ears can make no sense of sound. Communication, like food, is sustenance, a staff of life for the once-integrated person.

As words from members of my family, my friends, chance acquaintances receded, as they diminished to whispers and as my hearing further disintegrated, faded completely, I felt deserted by the hearing world. Profound hunger to understand the spoken word, profound frustration, profound anger took over. Surrounded by silence, I turned my hearing aids too high. I elevated my telephone amplifier excessively. Silence became raucous distortion.

There had to be a calm meeting with all the fears that beset people with hearing loss. As my hearing disability progressed from severe to very severe, I made this decision and I talked with many other hearing-impaired people, in all walks of life, who made the same decision.

Actor Michael Higgins

When I interviewed Michael Higgins, he explained that he was already a professional actor when he became hearing impaired. An active member of New York Circle Repertory Company, he appeared in the world premieres of Lanford Wilson's *A Tale Told* and Timothy Mason's *Levitation*. He received the acclaim of New York critics for performances in *The Sea Gull, Love's Labour Lost,* and *The Iceman Cometh* and won an Obie as the father in *Reunion.* On Broadway he starred with Julie Harris and Geraldine Page in *Mixed Couples, Whose Life Is It Anyway?* and *Equus.* Among his long list of credits and awards are nominations for Best Actor and Best Supporting Actor by the National Society of Film Critics and raves for his roles in *Wanda, The Conversation, The Black Stallion, Fort Apache-The Bronx* and Horton Foote's *1918.*

Michael Higgins told me how he refused to let his hearing impairment get in the way of his career.

"When I was a platoon leader in Italy, in World War II, I sustained a severe head wound in combat. More than a hearing problem, I developed a comprehension problem. At first I thought it was just a hearing deficiency, but then I realized things didn't make sense and I kept losing contact in group conversations. This added weight to my hearing loss. I realized I had to avoid complicated situations, complicated language. This became quite a problem in my acting career.

"Sentences would become convoluted in my mind. When listening to words on stage and working in film, the hearing loss and my bad comprehension overlapped. I first had to learn not to let this problem overwhelm me if I was to continue with my career.

"The best situations for me were scenes with just a few characters. When there were many people on stage at one time, I had to rehearse with very strong, focused concentration. This produced a great drain on my energy, but I understood my problem a little better and was able to carry on with my career. By keeping the working script with me day and night (even long before the first rehearsals, if possible) I was able to keep up with the progress of the work. It was a constant adjustment to situations. Listening! Listening!

"Doing a play is very precise work. You have to come in on cue and speak on cue. I prepare for the worst and think for the best.

"I never thought of abandoning my profession. I went to school at the American Theater Wing Professional Training Program for four years after I got out of the army, all the time working actively on Broadway. When problems would arise, I made myself overlook them so I could get on with what I could do. I wanted to be an actor all my life and wasn't going to let a head wound stop me.

"When I looked for employment, there was difficulty when people spoke too quietly or too rapidly. I needed time to grasp the sense of what was being said. I would sell myself by saying, 'Just let me read the part. Let me show you I can do it.'

"In interviews, especially for jobs for the movies, there is a lot of small talk. This is usually very difficult for me to follow because people doing the hiring will jump from one subject to another, losing me. I would still be trying to keep up with the first subject, and they'd already be on subject number three. I couldn't say, 'Wait a minute, you're jumping all over the place.' I would just try to make some sense of what was being said. Selling myself, getting the job, is always the hardest part.

"When I work, I direct myself to concentrate on the play. Nothing must interfere with the way I do my part, with the words I am to speak. The tremendous frustration is when I cannot hear. If I cannot hear another actor, I cannot hear the communication.

"I've had to learn to adjust to the hearing problem I have, the tinnitus, and the lack of comprehension due to my shrapnel head wound. I have to concentrate tremendously to see what other actors are doing as we rehearse and to keep things spontaneous.

"Initial interviews, of course, are more difficult. I don't know how people will talk. I don't know what to expect. The people interviewing me are often meeting me for the first time; watching me trying to adjust to a script I know nothing about; seeing me overalert, trying to focus, rather than being easy. They are not seeing me the way I would normally do the character on stage.

"When I can, I ask the casting people if I can see the script beforehand, even take it home to study. After all, they are interested in me as an actor, how I read the script, not in the interview. 'Forget the interview,' I would like to say. 'Let me read the script, let me study it.' Often, of course, you can't get to that point. But if I do get the script in advance of the reading, the audition goes well, without problems.

"One thing is true. When you have a deficit, hearing in my case, you become aware that most everybody has some problem. We just have to use our energy to overcome these problems in the most positive and natural way we can. There's a lot of emotion here. I find my perception of emotions has become greater because of my hearing loss. I can see people's emotions very clearly, without words, which is very important in the theater because theater has so much to do with emotions and feelings. I can tell when people are cheating on the stage, when they are not true. It is more than the hearing. Their faces, their body movements, tell me what they are feeling, what they are reacting to.

"If you look at two people on the street who are involved in an exchange that is obviously emotional, you know—without hearing them—what is going on by looking at their faces. You sense their feelings. You may not know the situation, but you sense what is going on. With hearing impairment you have to learn to substitute vision for hearing. It's a natural substitute. By constantly going out rather than going inward, hearing-impaired people learn to naturally pick up things that people with normal hearing don't usually sense. That's a big plus."

* * *

How people with hearing impairment fear becoming disconnected from former lives! Michael Higgins made the adjustment, holding on to what he once had. Others are less fortunate. My friend Cynthia fell apart when hearing impairment forced her to leave the teaching profession. The trauma of being set out to pasture, of no longer spending her days with young people, whom she took such great pleasure in nurturing with daily events to clue them into the environment of history that would determine their future, made her feel like a nonperson. Indeed, she did become a dropout for a while.

Lawyer Trudie Katz Walker

How does a lawyer, also dependent upon hearing words, words that could affect the lives of clients, manage when impairment of the auditory sense occurs?

The disconnection is traumatic when it happens to a person with an already established career. But here, at least, there is background, something of substance to lean on. In the case of Trudie Katz Walker, a young girl when her hearing became impaired, the disconnection was from a dream, a childhood aspiration to become a lawyer. To refuse this disconnection was exceedingly brave and daring. Lawyer Trudie Katz Walker tells her story:

"I have a hereditary sensorineural hearing loss. The problem comes from my mother's father's side of the family. We have traced members of the family with hearing loss back to cousins in Europe. Our family problem is a slow, degenerative condition with marked losses triggered by physical and hormonal changes.

"As a child of eight or nine, I was already showing some marked loss. It accelerated because I was highly allergic. In bad allergy seasons my hearing loss was worse.

"I really had no functional disability until near the end of college. At about age twenty, I noticed some severe problems. I had a very bad case of the flu that furthered the severity. At that point I realized I was having difficulty, and I went for more tests. When I recovered from the flu, my hearing condition cleared up somewhat, and I decided to ignore it.

"My mother went to the same doctor a short time later and the doctor said, 'Why hasn't your daughter come back to take care of her hearing problem?'

"My mother has the same condition; however, her loss is not as great as mine. Hers did not become acute until she reached the age of fifty. Her loss was in combination with her age loss, which is a common occurrence for many people. Age loss plus menopausal hormonal changes. This is when she suffered an acute loss. My sister also has a loss; however, there is no evidence of loss in our children as yet.

"I realized I could not attend law school and sit in classrooms without a hearing aid. So at twenty-three I entered law school and started to wear a hearing aid. But I still fought it and would not wear my hearing aid except in a classroom situation. When I attended classes at law school, I would request to be seated up front. My condition is degenerative, and over a period of time I constantly lost more hearing.

"In my social life I had no difficulties, no problems dating, no social rejection that I was aware of. After I was married and started to practice law, I began to wear a second hearing aid, although I should have been using a second aid a lot sooner.

"During pregnancy I suffered a tremendous additional hearing loss. Because of the nature of my condition, the loss is hormonally triggered. I suffered this very large loss in my sixth week of pregnancy, almost overnight. My hearing has further deteriorated the last five years, and I notice much more functional difficulty.

"I taught college many years and found that I had tremendous difficulty with my students. But I found most of the students to be extremely cooperative when I came forward with my hearing loss. I requested changes to rooms that were acoustically better than others. To some extent, I was given courtesy of room changes.

"Professionally, I have been able to manage well with my hearing loss. In court I have never been denied a seat near the bench. At conferences seating is arranged to accommodate my problem. I'm not concerned about asking a judge to repeat something. I'm very open; I put it up front and tell everybody they have to look at me when they speak and enunciate clearly.

"The greatest difficulty I have is when I'm nervous. When I'm nervous, I don't synthesize as rapidly as when I'm relaxed. This is where I have my biggest problem professionally. My other major problem is with telephone equipment. AT&T is best for me. However, some of their newer telephone equipment does not work as well as their original amplified handset.

"I've never had formal training in speechreading, and I cannot depend wholly on speechreading. When someone has a beard or mustache, I'm at a severe disadvantage because I cannot see their mouth forming words. Multiparty conferences are very difficult because I'm not in a position to look at everyone while conversation goes on around a large conference table. But I have found that people are usually very cooperative.

"Some social settings are very difficult for me. Dinner with several couples in a restaurant—forget it! I can't understand a thing. I might as well not be there. Background noise in restaurants makes understanding impossible.

"Defining relationships within my family in terms of my hearing impairment, I have to say my son, who is five years old, is terrific. My husband is the difficult one. He is not a loud or a clear talker. I sometimes call him 'marble mouth.' He doesn't attempt to enunciate clearly and for many years, in my opinion, was rather inconsiderate for not making the necessary effort. He has improved, though, particularly when he has to talk to me on the telephone. But he doesn't speak clearly automatically. My son, on the other hand, is fantastic. He looks directly at me when he talks and never gets angry or impatient when he has to repeat something.

"My son tells his friends, 'My mommy is special. You're supposed to look at her when you talk.' My son is just wonderful. His speech is very clear and has been from the day that he started to talk. I do, however, have difficulty with other children in my son's kindergarten set. Many do not speak clearly and when they come to play at my house, I do have some difficulty. If the little ones have colds or sound nasal, I'm lost. But my son will interpret for me.

"In the practice of law I've never had a problem with clients being unwilling to work with me because of my hearing problem. As a young attorney I encountered more problems being a female in the profession than in being hearing impaired. But, of course, hearing impairment makes my work more difficult. I'm much more tired at the end of the day than I would be if I were not impaired.

"I've never had a negative reaction from the bench. I've always had cooperation. Though I do have to remind judges, from time to time, that I have a hearing problem."

The Late Honorable Claude Pepper

There are many ways to hear: hear but not absorb; hear but not comprehend what is said; hear but not listen; hear but not care about what is said. A person with all sensory hair cells in mint condition may, in fact, make far less use of hearing than a person with severe hearing impairment.

Making positive use of society's vocabulary requires more than healthy sensory cells. When I interviewed the late Claude Pepper, I knew he had a gift more valuable than healthy ears: the gift of listening with an unselfish heart and soul. His constituents and the elderly for whom he was a folk hero—indeed, the entire country—profited immensely from the way this man wearing two hearing aids heard their language.

The Honorable Claude Pepper, octogenarian member of Congress, wore two hearing aids. He also wore a pacemaker and the scars of open-heart surgery. He worked 15 hours a day and traveled extensively from coast to coast. Claude Pepper, affectionately called "the Senator," talked about his experiences with hearing impairment, experiences that did not interfere with his long congressional career:

"My hearing loss started many years ago. At first it was not too bad. It was a gradual loss. My wife began to notice it at first. I was not quite hearing everything that was being said, and my wife suggested that I check my hearing to see if I needed a hearing aid. I took her good advice and found out that I was missing words and should get a hearing aid.

"At first I got the small hearing aids that fit into the ear. I wore them for a few years. Then, at Walter Reed Hospital, where I would take my hearing tests, I was told that those small aids were too weak for me. They recommended I get a different type of hearing aid with a larger battery, more powerful, to send a larger sound to the inner ear. I now have an aid for each ear. Most of the time I wear the two. Sometimes, though, I wear just one.

"I can get along pretty well using just one hearing aid unless I am in the Senate or House chamber or in a public meeting somewhere where the acoustics may not be good; then I do better with two. I can get along with one, but I generally wear two to get the best results. And I never have the slightest embarrassment. I know a lot of other people who wear hearing aids and have other defects. Now, I've been wearing glasses since I was forty years old. The glasses are just a supplement to help me see. And that's what a hearing aid is; it's just a supplement to hear. There is nothing more extraordinary about needing to wear a hearing aid than needing to wear glasses. So why be embarrassed? I went ahead and got the best hearing aids I could, and I used them as best I could.

"But I will say this. I think children should be taught to lipread. They never know when they will sustain a hearing loss. If they can lipread, they will be prepared for such a loss. They will be able to use a hearing aid better and understand more of what is being said. And if they learn to read lips, they will be more aware of people with hearing problems and they will speak more distinctly.

"If I'm in a crowd, say, at a cocktail party where there is a lot of noise and I am speaking to people at close range, I usually take the hearing aid out of my right ear.

This will cut off some of the other noises. I can hear better in a crowded, noisy place like that without the second hearing aid than with it. Especially if I am speaking to someone close by. I lean over very near to the person and let that individual speak to me directly. Ordinarily, without the hearing aid in my right ear, I can hear what he or she has to say. I don't have too many experiences with the individual who will smother his speech with his hands. But I will usually speak to one person directly who is close by.

"I like to tell a story that involves a misunderstanding because of hearing impairment. I told it in New York, where I was speaking to a group that was there for an Aging Conference. A couple came down to Miami to celebrate their fiftieth wedding anniversary. She was quite hard-of-hearing. They decided to stay a week, and they had a wonderful time living their romance all over again. Every day the husband told his wife several times, over and over—because she was hard-of-hearing and could miss some of his words—how much he loved her, how wonderful she was, and what it had meant to him to be her husband for half a century.

"Finally, it was the last day of their trip. They were lunching in a restaurant that looked out over Biscayne Bay. He was sitting on one side of the table and she on the other. He looked and saw the palms waving in the breeze and the whitecaps bending on the sea. With the loveliness of the scene out there, romance came once more to his lips, and he thought one more time he would tell his wife how much he loved her. Looking directly across the table to her he said, 'Very honestly, I'm proud of you.' She looked back at him and said, 'And, very honestly, I'm tired of you too.'

"This story gets a good laugh. I hear a lot of stories like this about not hearing correctly. This can be a subject for laughter. I mean, to some people. But generally the inability to hear is not a funny thing, it is a regrettable thing. But until they find some way to overcome it, other than by wearing hearing aids, I don't know anything to do but use the aids we now have and go on the best we can.

"I never thought my hearing impairment might interfere with my legislative career. I felt I could just use hearing aids to get along. Frequently, I speak before audiences. I hear them quite well if they have something to say, and I can hear quite well when I am introduced. Difficulty I have is in a big chamber or if I'm with people who don't speak distinctly. One Sunday night I was one of the speakers in a forum for the elderly in New York. I could hear some of the speakers, and there were some I could not hear. What I did was adjust my hearing aids for each speaker. For some speakers I had too much power on, so I lowered it a little. For other speakers I had to increase the power. Generally, I get along satisfactorily.

"I am chairman of a very important committee. Sometimes I have to ask people on the committee to repeat what they said. There is no harm or embarrassment about asking people to repeat something.

"My hearing loss does not keep me from traveling a lot and working very long hours. I have the strength to do all these things. Every now and then I do have a little cold or a touch of the flu, which can slow me down a bit, but normally I'm very active. I walk faster than most people who walk with me. I'm alert when I work with my staff. I can pick up a sentiment and dictate a little speech in just minutes. I've been fortunate to have vigor and vitality to carry a heavy work load without feeling burdened. In my younger years I was never tired. Now, I'm sometimes a little tired when I get home. I just lie down on my bed for a while until I get refreshed, and then I get up to read or watch television.

"I'm called upon by many different size groups. One had thirty or forty people with former Senator Tydings in one of the rooms at the Capitol. They had gotten together to help each other with private business. I made a little speech to them.

"This past Sunday night, at an Aging meeting in New York, there were people from all over the world. A lady asked me to speak at an Elderly Fair in Philadelphia. I speak all over the country and my hearing loss is not a problem.

"But I'd like to get back to the subject of children learning to lipread. I feel very strongly about this. It would be the wise thing to do. Children can easily be taught to lipread in school. This should not wait until they reach my age, when there is often hearing difficulty.

"People tell me that to understand the meaning of what is being said, just look at lips. It is true that if you look at lips you get a lot of help. But if you have learned this skill as a child, it would be much easier. You'd be prepared should you develop impaired hearing.

"Children should also be taught to speak clearly. Mothers should say, 'Get that gum out of your mouth, please. Speak so that we can understand you. Don't slur your speech.' It might be a good idea for mothers to conduct these lessons at the dining table.

"The main thing is to not put off getting hearing aids when they are needed. Not to suffer the deprivation of that available benefit. Adjust yourself, help yourself as best you can against a health impediment.

"I'm always making adjustments. During legislative sessions and public hearings in congressional chambers I listen very intently. If I need to, I can walk around and sit down right in front of the speaker. One usually speaks at the table down front of the Speaker of the House in what we call the well of the House. And I can sit down right behind or right in front of the speaker and be close by.

"But I usually sit at a place that's at the end of a table. I used to sit there nearly all the time, and, you know, we habituate ourselves as to where we sit. But I make adjustments to hear correctly. Sometimes I'll ask other members, 'What was that last point he or she made? I'm not sure I got it.' Sometimes there is laughter, and I'll ask other members, 'What was that point of humor? I didn't get it.' I may miss some humor or some words I would like to hear, but this does not interfere with my understanding of what is being said in the main. It doesn't interfere with the performance of my work.

"Even though I am elected by and work for the people of Florida's Eighteenth District, I regard all the people from all districts as my concern. I'm constantly concerned with the public good, things that are best for, in the best interest of, people generally, all over the country.

"I just want to add this: Hearing impairment is one of the impediments which comes along in life. Sometimes it comes along early in life, through an accident or such. Sometimes it comes with aging. We should accept it with equanimity when it comes. Not lose our poise, not lose our high purpose. We should make the effort to alleviate it or diminish it and keep on with our face towards the east, marching into the sun. We should not be discouraged. Make the best of what the Lord allows us and keep going and doing."

Financial Executive Gary McKae

Hearing-disabled people are always part of each other's lives. When I talked with Gary McKae, sales manager of the Merrill Lynch San Francisco office, his simple truths, unlike my own, still were mine. With deep emotion, he spoke about awakening from coma to discover his deafness, likening the event to a Fellini film:

"My hearing impairment started in 1978. I was with Bache and Company in Hawaii at the time. I was attending a meeting of the Financial Planners Association in Chicago, and I had no hearing impairment. At a seminar, listening to a speaker, I began feeling ill. I had a terrible headache and began sweating, so I went to a colleague's room in the hotel.

"The next thing I remember was opening my eyes—I didn't realize I'd been in a coma—and feeling as though I was in a Fellini film. It seemed to me that I was looking up through a funnel. The room was all white. Machines were over my head, and a priest was giving me my last rites. My comment was, 'What the fuck am I doing here!'

"Then everything faded away. A nurse and doctor were in front of me. They were speaking to me, but I didn't hear anything being said. I told them, 'I can't hear a word you're saying.' They continued talking, and I became very upset and said, 'Damn it! I can't hear you.'

"This scene kept fading in and out. Next, the doctor was writing, and he showed me a note that read YOU ARE DEAF. AND WE DON'T KNOW WHY.

"For a long time I was in intensive care, on IV and machines. There were spinal taps. The doctor wrote on a piece of paper YOU HAVE SPINAL MENINGITIS AND WE DON'T KNOW IF YOU'RE GOING TO MAKE IT. As though it happened yesterday, I remember saying, 'I'm in your hands and in the hands of a person greater than you.'

"I kept going into and coming out of comas. I remember waking up once and having part of my hearing back, although everything I heard people saying sounded like Mickey Mouse or Donald Duck. For about a month I was in intensive care in Resurrection Hospital in Chicago.

"I had a number of hearing tests. Dr. José Ferrer— who looked very much like José Ferrer—said to me, 'You've lost more than fifty percent of your hearing, and we doubt if you will hear more than that anymore.'

"This loss has been very difficult from the standpoint of common things in life I could no longer hear—telephones ringing, teapots boiling. When I came home, I could not understand what my children were saying to me. They were very young girls with delicate voices. I could hear their voices but couldn't understand what they said.

"I took many hearing tests and found that I had lost all the upper frequencies. I went to a number of specialists. My home at the time was Honolulu. I was very frustrated and, for a time, did nothing but walk from my bed to a couch. When my little girls lay on my stomach and hugged me, it pained me that I could not understand what they were saying. I was unable to talk with people over the telephone. When I began walking out of doors, there was the pain of living in Hawaii and not being able to hear the ocean roar, not hearing a bird.

"After about six months I went back to work as a broker. One of my clients was a physician. He told me, 'I'm not a hearing specialist. I'm a general practitioner. I've been playing around with acupuncture.'

"He suggested we try something the Chinese use called homeopathic acupuncture. This involved taking various solutions and injecting them into my hearing points on an acupuncture basis. He thought this might give me the chance of getting part of my hearing back.

"This was happening at a very bad time in my life. My wife had become despondent. We had lost most of our net worth. She began drinking a lot and blamed me for her problem.

"I let the doctor do this acupuncture for about a year and a half. Eventually, I got all but thirty percent of my hearing back. What I have is nerve deafness. The doctor told me it was not the meningitis that gave me the deafness, it was the medication I was on when I had the meningitis. The medication I was on was ampicillin.

"I use amplifiers in my telephone and I use hearing aids. The hearing aids help somewhat but also make problems. They make noises in the background much louder, so this noise can often overpower the person talking next to me. I realize I have my limitations and have to live with them.

"I've learned to read lips though I'm not an excellent lipreader.

"When Bache was bought out by Prudential, I went to A G Becker. When they were bought out, I became the manager of an institutional house. When they were bought out, I went back to Merrill Lynch, where I had started in 1970.

"I am six foot three, two hundred and twenty pounds, and in the best of physical shape, so it's hard for me to think of myself as disabled. I had to deal with this the first few years of my hearing disability. The fact is, I am disabled and not all firms I've been with could accommodate my disability. Even at Merrill Lynch, where my disability is understood, there is a long way to go in dealing with a hard-of-hearing employee. The business environment is a one-hundred-percent hearing environment. During seminars and at training sessions I sit up front, work hard at listening, and hope there will be enough reading material. I always miss something, which I accept, and just do the best I can. I'm not only dealing with a hearing environment, but I also have to deal with lack of understanding and prejudice in this environment. I think, as a result, I have a better understanding of other disabled people, of prejudices and frustrations, of all minority problems. I'm more empathetic than I was before my disability.

"I've become a face-to-face person, which helps in dealing with clients, and I've been extremely successful. I concentrate more keenly than I did before my hearing loss. In this sense my disability has been a big plus for my business.

"Of course, I've run into problems that all hearing-impaired people must run into. When I was at the Merrill Lynch Assessment Center, in group sessions four or five people would talk at once and I would be lost. I'm also lost at cocktail parties. I might just as well sit in a corner with a glass in my hand. At the first cocktail party I went to after my illness, I didn't know what was going on. In frustration, I sat by myself and drank until I was absolutely soused.

"I'm very fortunate that there are wonderful people in my life who come to my aid when I need it. My new wife is very understanding, and she is a big help to me at social functions. And I have a great assistant at Merrill Lynch. She comes to my rescue when I cannot understand a voice on the telephone or when people talk to me without facing me. She puts lots of things in writing to make sure I understand what is going on. And then there are my wonderful, loving daughters. I'm also fortunate that the words *buy* and *sell* look so different and sound so different. Knock on wood, I haven't made errors.

"In my present position I'm a producing sales manager, which means I'm also a financial consultant or broker. As sales manager I deal with eighty brokers. At sales meetings I can't hear questions from the back of the room, and I don't always know what is being said. My assistant is a big help.

"Merrill Lynch has a special program for the hearing-impaired and deaf. It is probably the greatest service that an investment firm could put together. The company realized that there are people out there who have a distinct disability that is not visible and set out to establish a network of financial consultants around the country to serve the financial needs of the millions of hearing-impaired people. TDDs (telecommunication device for the deaf, now called text telephone, or TTY) are used to communicate with the deaf and very hearing-impaired through a typewriter/telephone. I'm not aware of any other investment firm with this kind of program.

"But even this kind of program can't completely answer the pain of hearing impairment. In the end, it's up to the individual to develop the right attitude. During one of my very low times, emotionally low times, I met a broker who was in a wheelchair. He told me he had an automobile accident when he was twenty-four—when I met him he was fifty-four—and he talked about things he used to love doing: golf, running, swimming, surfing. He said at least he'd been able to enjoy those things, unlike someone who was born with his disability.

"I realized I too was fortunate at least to have the memory of birds singing and the ocean roaring. So I count my blessings for what I have known, or have heard, and for all the things I can still do now."

Chapter 10

Bodybuilder and Football Star

The Incredible Hulk, Lou Ferrigno

I think meeting Lou Ferrigno, who knew the pain of hearing impairment as a child and learned to live with it, making a fine career as a bodybuilder and another in films as the Incredible Hulk, was a turning point for me. If Lou Ferrigno could make his way so successfully among the hearing, why not me? Why not all people with hearing disorders?

In an interview Ferrigno told me his inspiring story:

"When I was three years old I had bad ear infections that caused me to lose between seventy and seventy-five percent of my hearing. My parents took me to many, many doctors. The very best doctors. By the time I was four years old, I was fitted with hearing aids. I can remember that my mother cried the first time she put the earmold into my ears.

"I don't remember how words sounded to me when my hearing first became damaged. But I do remember being quite curious about the little molds my mother would put into my ears and about the part of the old-fashioned apparatus that was strapped to my chest. By the time I went off to school, I had to learn to use the aids myself. I had to learn how to put new batteries in when the ones I had in went dead. I didn't like to do this when the other kids could see. It was embarrassing.

"The other kids were pretty aware of the strange gadget I had to wear strapped to my chest. Sometimes they tried to grab the strap off my chest. It certainly wasn't a very easy situation. They would also call me by unpleasant names. 'Deaf Louie,' they'd shout at me. Or 'Tin ear.' Sometimes they'd call me 'the mute.' It was no fun. I was always afraid they would ruin my hearing aid. And I was always worried the batteries would go dead. And when they did go dead, I would just pretend that I could hear what kids were saying. But of course I could not understand what they were saying. So I would pretend. Those were not at all happy times.

"I guess because I wasn't a fighter, it was easy for other kids to take advantage of me, of my problem with hearing. I soon found ways to enjoy being by myself. I guess you might say I found an escape. I escaped with comic books. My father was a policeman. We weren't rich, but we were comfortable. My father was sad that I was a loner, but he bought me all the comic books he could find. Those were my happy times, reading about Superman and the Incredible Hulk. I could read about them and pretend they were my friends or that I was like them and could perform superhuman tasks. So when other kids were not being friendly, when they were running after me and calling me Deaf Louie, I was able to stay cool and escape to my comic book heroes.

"I found another way to escape also. I started body-building. My father kept himself fit with some weights, and I decided to try them. I guess I was around eleven or twelve when I was using my father's weights pretty well. This gave me a lot of confidence. I could get along without those kids who weren't too nice. I developed self-admiration and self-respect watching myself lifting weights. My father helped me set up a long mirror in our basement where I lifted weights, and I could see myself developing. This is how I was able to stop caring what kids called me. It didn't matter so much what they said or thought about me. I was learning to believe in myself.

"Of course, I did have a few friends. Kids who were kind and understanding. And this was very vital to me. But this happened later on. Not when I was very young. In a way, maybe it was my fault too. Maybe I wasn't very likable because I was so introverted. But getting into bodybuilding was what changed that. Lifting weights and bodybuilding gave me self-confidence, so I was able to make some friends and things got better. Having friends who liked me in spite of my problem, having friends who understood me, was very helpful.

"When I think back about my school experiences, I blame myself for some of my difficulties. I was just too shy. There were teachers who would have helped me. They didn't know I had a hearing problem at the beginning of the term. I spoke poorly because I didn't hear words correctly enough to learn to imitate them correctly, and I insisted to my teachers that I had a speech problem, not a hearing problem. I didn't want teachers or anyone to know about my hearing problem.

"I didn't want people pitying me. I didn't want sympathy. It embarrassed me. And I didn't know how to explain my hearing problem so that I wouldn't get pity. I didn't know enough to just ask for help. I stayed shyly at the back of the room in school and pretended to hear what was going on. Wearing hearing aids doesn't help you understand what is being said when you are all the way at the back of a room. The result was, I ended up flunking examinations. And then I would have to study very hard by myself to be able to pass at the end of the semester.

"What I did learn in school was mainly from books. Very hard work by myself with books. Unfortunately, most examinations were mainly based on classroom teaching, so I didn't do as well as I might have. Because I was so shy and fearful of being made fun of if my hearing problem were known, I missed out on a lot. I missed out on education, and I missed out on life. It took me a long time to learn that I better get up the courage to ask people to repeat something I could not hear well enough to understand.

"What finally happened during my school years was that my parents had to come to school and tell the teachers about my hearing problem. But that didn't make me feel very happy either. It would help with my classwork because I'd be given a seat right up front, but I still felt worried about making my hearing problem known. I guess a hearing problem is harder on a kid than an adult. It can be more humiliating. Like the time some kids pulled the hearing aid mold right out of my ear. Yanked it right out. I was afraid they broke it—and my father was a policeman, so we weren't rich—and that hearing equipment cost a lot of money. When kids did that and I told them how much money my hearing aids cost, they laughed. And that was even more upsetting. I'd be too upset to try to be reasonable with them. I just wanted to get through those growing-up days. I wanted to get through them somehow and build my body so that it would be very strong. And I thought someday those kids would want to be my friends.

"It's those kinds of experiences that make a child want to rush his childhood away. Why not? There is not enough enjoyment. Those kinds of things leave scars. But I overcame those scars with my bodybuilding.

"I spent too much time by myself when I was a kid. I read every comic book I could get my hands on. A lot of the Marvel comic books. I'd read and read and memorize the words and actions of characters like the Incredible Hulk and Superman. And when I was spending all that time by myself, I'd fantasize about living in the same world with Superman and the Incredible Hulk. Then I'd imagine myself big and strong and heroic. I spent so many hours a day reading about the heroes I wanted to be, reading and reading, my mother and father used to say to me, 'Louie, if you would spend half the time with your schoolwork and your schoolbooks, you could become a doctor.' And they were right. That was true. When I wasn't reading about my heroes, I was working out to become like my heroes. At first I was using my father's weights and equipment. But I soon enough wanted additional weights and more equipment. Better equipment, which I had to work for. What money I earned, what money was given to me on special occasions, I used to build my workout room in our basement. My father helped me do a lot of the building. My mother and my grandmother helped also. They made me the kind of food I told them I needed in order to develop the body I was hoping for.

"Lots of things happen that can make hearing impairment especially difficult for a child. One time when I was at camp when I was a little kid, we were playing hide-and-seek. It was my turn to close my eyes while the other kids went to hide. What happened then was, my hearing aid battery went dead. I didn't have another battery with me. I wandered and wandered, trying to find the other kids. But because I couldn't hear any footsteps, it was very difficult to know where to look.

"I didn't even know what direction they took. I couldn't hear the whispering or laughing they might be doing. I couldn't hear anything to give me a clue about which way they went. I should have called out to them but I didn't like to admit to my hearing problem. I just wanted to be like the other kids and play the game like they played it. So I kept wandering and wandering, and I got deeper and deeper into the woods. Soon I was very lost. And then it got to be dark. There I was, lost in a dark woods without any hearing. I called out a little, but then I stopped because I was even too frightened to call or to cry. By the time I was found by some strange people, not by people from the camp, I was chilled as well as terribly frightened. My speech wasn't too good at the time, and I think they thought I was retarded. I couldn't hear what they said or what they asked me, but I could tell by the way they looked at me they thought something was wrong with me. I thought if I told them I didn't hear and couldn't speak well because of my hearing, they'd think plenty was wrong with me. But soon I did make them understand. I was certainly relieved to be found, but I still didn't like talking about my hearing problem. I didn't learn enough from that terrible experience.

"I knew for a long time that because I didn't hear words the right way, I was having trouble imitating them correctly. But I really became aware of my speech problem and aware that I had better do something about it when I won the Mr. Universe competition. I was twenty-one years old then. After I won the competition, they filmed an interview with me. It was supposed to be on television, but they couldn't use it because they felt that my speech was just not clear enough to be understood. Until then I was my own speech pathologist. But after that big disappointment, I decided to take speech lessons and really improve my speech.

"I had to start admitting to my hearing problem at the time I began doing the Incredible Hulk series. People I worked with thought I was drunk or stupid because of the way I spoke. Now this goes back many years. Today they don't think that anymore. I knew then I had to talk up about my hearing problem. I elaborated on the fact that I had a hearing problem. A lot of people in Hollywood assumed the wrong ideas, thought the wrong things about me at first. But once I explained about my hearing being impaired since I was a small child, things got better. Now, I'm well accepted. Of course, with speech lessons my speech got so much better too that the old speech problems are hardly noticeable.

"Another thing that makes it important to tell people about your hearing impairment is that then you have a better relationship. I've had some funny experiences. Sometimes I hear a word wrong and then I catch myself— or someone will tell me something that makes me know I heard wrong—and I will be able to laugh at myself. I can share my mistake with friends, and we can laugh together.

"Being a hearing-impaired actor, you have to be alert at every moment. It is very important that you study the script exceptionally well. You really have to do more work than a hearing actor to be sure you don't miss a cue. I rarely miss a cue because I stay so alert. But on the other hand, being hearing impaired, I learned a lot that helped me with my acting. When I watched television when I was a kid, I couldn't hear the words; so I would stare at the faces. This taught me to read emotions without words, and it taught me how to act out emotions so they could be read even though I didn't speak. This knowledge was very helpful because in the beginning my roles had no words. The Incredible Hulk just acted without words. And I used what I learned to show through body language alone what the Incredible Hulk was thinking and what he was feeling. This knowledge of making your body talk without words was also helpful when I competed in bodybuilding contests. In bodybuilding, they judge you on your body movements, not on your hearing and speech. It is all in body motion. In body emotion.

"In acting the Incredible Hulk, I was able to show the great sensitivity I have in my character because of all the sad problems I had with my hearing impairment. My hearing loss made me unique in that way, in that character role, and it came through, even through all that makeup.

"When I was asked to audition for the role of the Hulk and I went down for the screen test, they liked the way I showed my emotions without speaking. So that changed my whole life. I did not find it too difficult to make the transition from a professional bodybuilder to an actor. Performing as a bodybuilder was a great help to me in portraying the Hulk. Also, I knew the Hulk very well, since my childhood of reading comic books. In a way I had been preparing for this role for years and years. It was like a dream really come true.

"I had many things to overcome because of my hearing impairment. I was too shy to date girls until I got out to California with my bodybuilding and then my acting. But I did get up the courage to meet my beautiful wife, and I have a beautiful daughter and two fine little sons. The adjustments they have to make are not very easy. At times I may not be wearing any hearing aids and I am not able to hear them at all at those times, and that can be frustrating for them. They usually work twice as hard as other wives and children in order to handle my problem, and this is not very easy on a relationship or on the family itself. Even when I do wear my hearing aids, don't forget, I do not always hear as well as other people do, so it requires more patience on the part of my family than is required on the part of a family of a man who does have his normal hearing. Then too they are not always sure I have heard or heard correctly, and that is another strain.

"For people married to someone with hearing impairment, I have some helpful thoughts: Be patient and understanding. Talk slowly and go into detail carefully. My wife sometimes forgets to do this. Going into detail is extremely important. If the person who can hear gives a message to a person who has hearing trouble and gives a fast summary of what he or she thinks is the important part of the message, a detail may be left out which could be essential to the hearing-impaired person. Because each of us interprets things differently. What may seem an unimportant aspect to one may be the key to another. By leaving out certain details, mistakes and misunderstandings can happen. And that can result in much more lost time than if the mate took the time to tell all the details. It can also result in embarrassment and other problems.

"I have a message for hearing-impaired people who are too shy or embarrassed or too fearful to take advantage of all the help they could be getting either with hearing aids or with surgery: Don't hide away with your hearing problems. You only suffer in the long run. Don't put off getting help. Be sure to get competent help, though. And don't feel sorry for yourself. No one else is supposed to hold your hand and take care of you. Only you can do it for yourself. If you don't do what you can to help yourself, you are the one who pays the price. Stand up on your own two feet, and then you will appreciate yourself and so will other people appreciate you. There is plenty of help around, so don't be a quitter."

Larry Brown, Washington Redskins Running Back

I took the Williams Sound System with me for my interview with Larry Brown, Hall of Fame Washington Redskins running back. But assistive devices, other than my hearing aids, were unnecessary. He spoke so carefully that I had no difficulty understanding everything he told me about his experiences with hearing impairment:

"The first person to recognize that I had a real hearing problem was Vince Lombardi. That was in 1969. It was after reviewing several games and practice films that he noticed I was getting off the ball a split second later than everybody. He asked me about it, and I told him that I was a little hesitant in starting because I was having trouble reading the defensive alignment. That sat well with him for about a week. And then I guess after continuing to study the practice films, he noticed no significant

change. He decided—*without* my approval—to bring in a
hearing specialist, and he had me examined. This perhaps
confirmed his thought that I was totally deaf in my right
ear. And he was right. I am totally deaf in my right ear. It
has been explained to me by people in the hearing field
that I have a nerve-damaged right ear. To my knowledge, I
was born that way. I hear well out of my other ear, and
I've learned to compensate. When I was growing up, I
positioned myself in the right place, and I learned how to
read lips.

"If anyone knew about my deafness when I was a very
young child they never said anything. It was as an older
child that I realized I had some problem with my right ear.
Probably out of fear of being ridiculed or being looked
upon as being weird, I chose not to bring the matter up.
But I guess as I became a teenager, my mother and I
discussed my problem—though I never made it public
knowledge. I thought the best way to deal with it was not
to mention it if I wasn't asked about it.

"When voices were directed at my right ear, I was not
hearing them. I would turn my head in the direction of
where voices came from. But I would get in trouble when
there was enormous sound on my good side and I found
myself speaking to someone on my right. Then my hearing capabilities on my left were blocked.

"I would then depend on reading lips or pretend I was
understanding when I was not. The bottom line was that I
had problems. In a theater when someone sat at my right,
I could not hear that person. Wherever I was, if I was
listening to someone at the side of my good ear and someone tried speaking to me from the other side, I'd have a
serious problem. I never discussed the problem with
teachers or classmates.

"I recall taking hearing examinations somewhere in el-
ementary school, but no one ever said I was deaf in one
ear. Probably no one took enough interest in me to find
out what was wrong. I think I lost a good amount of edu-

cation along the way, especially in English classes, where paying close attention to the sounds of words was a big problem.

"Growing up, I must have heard lots of things incorrectly, which caused me problems along the way. I didn't participate in class discussions because I was shy and thought if I talked on some question, someone might realize I hadn't heard the question correctly.

"No one ever teased me about my hearing problem. Only very close friends knew about it, and they just accepted it. But there were always obstacles to overcome. I grew up in a ghetto of Pittsburgh where you might succumb to drugs or crime. I was small for someone who wanted to be a football player. I had a sinus condition that required two operations. I had knee injuries and a broken wrist. I was almost always in pain. And compounding this, there was the hearing problem.

"But I always set high goals in life. I realized that to get from point A to Z, even with good financial circumstances in a good environment, people still have problems. Of course, in my environment problems were magnified. I had to come a longer way and work harder. I always felt I could do anything I wanted to do, that the only thing that could stop me would be the lack of desire to succeed and excel. Whenever people tell me I can't do something, that gets my adrenalin flowing. I always challenge those people to prove they are wrong and I am right, based on performance, not lip service.

"When I was at Dodge City Community College and later at Kansas State, I was still concealing my hearing impairment from teammates and coaches. Throughout my athletic career, at the high school level and at college level, no one ever spoke about it. I just happened to be in the right places at the right times to hear enough correctly.

"Because of my hearing problem, I used to spend a lot of extra time reading and studying the information given me to make sure I understood it. Also, I was fortunate I had excellent recall. You need that, especially when you have a numerical play-calling system, play identification. In order to have a career, you have to have performances that are pretty much error-free.

"But concealing a hearing problem causes an extra burden and more hardship than admitting to it. You miss a lot along the way. Education is a sort of food for success. You need a good, solid education to be able to move into the marketplace and carve out your niche, to get a good job that will enable you to build a foundation for yourself. With my hearing problem going unnoticed, I was at risk. That was the main reason, when I first came to Washington, with the assistance of Vince Lombardi, I chose to go public and deal with my problem. There are probably many young people out there growing up as I did in fear of being exposed as having a hearing problem and losing a great deal of good information and education.

"There are always hardships. You just determine to get up and get there anyway. One time I injured an arm, and the injury required twenty stitches. The other players watching the doctor stitch up my arm seemed to be suffering more than I was. A doctor once told me I had a tremendous threshold or tolerance for pain. Maybe I trained myself this way. Like self-hypnosis. I conditioned myself to survive the years of growing up as a black child in a society that isn't always kind to its minorities. In other words, since I had a great deal to overcome in order to make my way, hearing impairment was just one more obstacle. So I learned when I was very young not to complain and not to look for help outside myself.

"Since high school I was a very independent person. I never wanted to cry or complain. That's developing a tolerance for pain. If I had problems, I'd focus on them and deal with them myself. I also felt that because other problems existed, like the treatment of minorities, I didn't want to compound those problems by letting my hearing problem surface.

"Sometimes problems make us stronger. You say to yourself, 'Well, I've conquered one, so I guess I can conquer the next.' Unfortunately, many young people go in an opposite direction. I think I coped so well because I had a wonderful mother and father, who helped give me inner strength. They were both very strong and very Christian, and they took a hard approach to help me recognize good from bad. My father is not alive now, but he did have the opportunity to see me play during the years of great attention and fanfare, the Super Bowl and such. My mother is still alive and comes down from Pittsburgh to Washington to visit with me every two weeks.

"When Vince Lombardi had a specialist confirm that I was hearing impaired, he wrote the commissioner of the National Football League, Pete Rozelle, and got permission to install a hearing aid in my helmet. The hearing aid was designed with a crossover technique: the hearing aid was on the side of my bad ear and would transmit sounds that came in on that bad side to my good ear. I don't believe it worked as well as people thought it would. A hearing aid is so delicate, and the punishment and pounding I was subjected to caused problems for the hearing aid. But I never told anyone. I just kept putting new batteries in it and never spoke about the constant bother. I wanted to cope with the problem by myself.

"The special hearing aid was taped inside my helmet. A cord ran through the suspension part of the helmet and was taped going right towards my opposite ear. It was like a telephone operator would have with a headset. Before every practice, before every game, I put in fresh batteries.

"After the special helmet, my game changed for the better. I wasn't getting off the ball late anymore, and I wasn't starting late anymore. Also, what helped me a great deal was the realignment. In the huddle, instead of facing the quarterback, I was put right next to the quarterback. This helped tremendously. Everything was super.

"There were some laughs along the way too. After I was examined by the hearing specialist, Vince Lombardi told me to put on the helmet that had been rigged up with the hearing aid. Then he sent me out to a far corner of the field. He shouted out to me, 'Larry, can you hear me?' I answered, 'Coach, nobody ever has a problem hearing *you*.' That got a good laugh.

"After my helmet was fitted with hearing equipment, I wanted to get fitted with something I could wear all the time. Unfortunately, there was nothing like that equipment for the helmet on the market, nothing with the crossover principle. Maybe I could have had that kind of wiring made to wear without a helmet, but I didn't want to go walking down the street with wires going around my head and down my neck. I had some glasses made with hearing aids attached. The hearing aid wires ran through the frames and through the rims. That worked pretty well for a while. But taking the glasses off and putting them on was hard on the wires. The sound soon got very distorted and the device began to malfunction. Then, two or three years later, this new technique came along. This device has two parts: one is the amplifier, and one is the receiver. These aids really work for people with my problem.

"The great Vince Lombardi was great for many reasons. He taught me more than the game of football. He taught me how to live with my problem. He gave me the confidence to get the help I needed.

"The hearing aid in my helmet was helpful for one very important play, probably my most important play, the play that gave me a thousand yards in a season for the first time. It was a moment in my life I look back on with joy and happiness.

"Having a hearing aid in my helmet certainly helped me in terms of getting a position on the team, having the opportunity to perform at a level that put me on the starting unit. If those two things had not occurred, then all the other important things that happened in terms of my contribution to the team and my rewards and recognition would never have occurred.

"Hearing signals clearly and the changing of signals is vital. Before the hearing aid setup in my helmet, it was like a guessing game. If I didn't hear the snap count in a huddle, I would wait until the center moved the ball to respond and start completing my responsibility and assignment. On the films, when they slow the film down, you can see me moving a split second after that ball moved. That's how Vince Lombardi detected my difficulty. That was one big problem I was having when they changed the play. It was not so much the play but the snap count, because I was at the other end of the huddle. When everybody broke out of the huddle and I did not hear the snap count, I compensated by just trying to move with the ball. But when they slowed the film, everything became obvious.

"I'm with Xerox now. My title is Business and Community Relations Manager, Mid-Atlantic Region. My responsibilities are to coordinate our employees' activities as they relate to community affairs and projects and to make decisions where Xerox presence is needed in the public.

"When I joined Xerox, I instituted a children's hospital fundraiser, which involved our marketing team in the sale of authentically autographed Washington Redskins footballs to our customers at five hundred dollars each. Mark Moseley agreed to be our cochairperson. This became an annual fundraising event. We now have fifty-two corporations involved.

"I've spoken to many hearing-impaired and deaf groups. One of my most interesting experiences was speaking at Gallaudet College. Someone stood next to me to interpret in sign what I said. There I was in this large room and the only sounds were plates and silverware. No voice except mine."

Aid for the Deaf Ear

Most people with one good ear and one profoundly deaf ear rely totally on the good ear to do all their hearing. Larry Brown did not accept this common notion and sought advice from Dr. Charles I. Berlin, Director of Louisiana State University Medical Center's Ear, Nose, and Throat Department's Kresge Hearing Research Laboratory of the South (New Orleans).

Dr. Berlin believes that two ears, no matter their condition, are better than one. He fitted Larry Brown's deaf ear with an aid that has the power to send vibrations through the skull to alert Brown's good ear that a message is coming in from an area in contact with his deaf ear.

When I interviewed Dr. Berlin, he talked about the research done in his laboratory by Dr. Webster: "Dr. Webster does research on the effect of hearing loss on brain anatomy, on what happens when you are deprived of hearing and the effect that has on brain growth and development. We have a feeling, more than scientific evidence, that using both sides of the brain is useful. There are animal systems that show if you don't stimulate both ears, then one side of the brain doesn't develop. But we have no real evidence that this is the case in humans. Only a suggestion of it. The most important thing is that we know that people hear better with two ears just as they see better with two eyes. Just as we would not wear a monocle or recommend one in our day except for very special situations.

"We recommend the use of two hearing aids because you hear better. You can detect where sound is coming from and can communicate far better in multiple conversations.

"We recommend two aids—but without any absolutely faultless scientific proof. That is the best and only way to go. The aid for Larry Brown was not original with me. I got the idea from an esteemed colleague, Dr. Roy Sullivan of Garden City, New York. It can be purchased on the commercial market. It is simply the application of a very powerful hearing aid being used in an otherwise nonresponsive ear to stimulate the bones of the skull."

When I discussed the importance of using two hearing aids with Dr. Joseph E. Hawkins, professor emeritus of otorhinolaryngology at the University of Michigan Medical School Kresge Hearing Research Institute in Ann Arbor, Michigan, he said "Binaural aids give one a better idea of auditory space. In addition, the two ears working together tend to cancel out some of the environmental noise."

I know from my own experience that two hearing aids are more than twice as good. For several years I resisted an aid for my ear with poorer discrimination. When I finally followed my audiologist's advice and began using a second aid, the improvement was incredible. I've been urging a second hearing aid on all my friends with two impaired ears who think one is enough. One is not nearly enough for people with hearing impairment who want the fullest communication with the hearing world.

Chapter 11

Beware the Pill

Medication and Hearing Loss

"I had only a slight hearing loss before I took those pills," my friend Cynthia told me. "Now I'm almost deaf."

Cynthia, as severely hearing impaired as I, was bitter that she could no longer teach at our local junior high school. She was bitter that her husband did not quite understand how to relate to a wife with severe hearing impairment, bitter that she had lost friends because severe hearing impairment limited the kind of socializing she could now do (the telephone chatting and so forth), bitter that her twin sons found talking with her a "drag." And she was particularly bitter that she had not been warned that diuretics might cause this adverse effect on her hearing.

Every day children and adults, placing trust in prescribers of pills, are jeopardizing their hearing. Dr. Christopher J. Linstrom, assistant director of otology at the New York Eye and Ear Infirmary, New York City, says, "Drugs are a two-edged sword. Antibiotic drugs and even a medication as common as aspirin, which is used in high doses for people with rheumatoid arthritis, are double-edged swords."

Dr. Robert E. Brummett, a leading ototoxicologist and professor of otolaryngology and pharmacology at Oregon Health Sciences University in Portland, says, "One thing about aspirin I am very suspicious of: that is, that it will produce tinnitus [ringing in the ear]. At the Tinnitus Clinic at the Oregon Research Center we have six or seven people with tinnitus that is reasonably permanent. And the only thing they have all had are very large doses of aspirin that caused the tinnitus acutely." Tinnitus can be a debilitating hearing disorder. Usually it is described as "ringing in the ear." However, tinnitus wears many hats. Some tinnitus sufferers say it is like the hissing of old-fashioned radiators. My friend Ralph says his tinnitus is like a waterfall. My friend Jean says she wishes her tinnitus sounded like a waterfall; her disorder is like a continuously whistling tea kettle. Beth thinks her tinnitus is the worst. She told me, "It's chirping, constant chirping that can make one suicidal." My neighbor Thelma's tinnitus produces noise like the motor of a jet plane. She will sometimes go to a crowded mall or department store where surrounding noises tend to cancel it out and give her a little relief from jet motors raging in her head. Inez carefully details her tinnitus: "It sometimes starts with a ticking noise, then I know it's coming. Buzzing starts like from a distance, then builds up to a crescendo, stops a second and repeats. Like a recording going on and on. During the day when I'm busy with chores, I can cope, but at night when I try to sleep, it's bad. If I manage to fall asleep when it's quiet, I can be awakened by loud buzzing. I rarely get a full night's sleep."

Across the country there are clinics to help people deal with tinnitus. And tinnitus victims are often unaware that aspirin may have gotten them there.

If an over-the-counter drug like aspirin can adversely affect the ear, what about the more potent prescription drugs? Dr. Leo Parmer, who was with the Food and Drug Administration for eight years, part of the time as deputy medical director, and who for nearly forty years has been chairperson of the Pharmacy and Therapeutics Committee at Long Island Jewish Medical Center in Queens, New York, says, "It is clear to me that most physicians are not completely familiar with the ototoxic effects of medications they are prescribing."

(*The Random House Dictionary of the English Language,* second edition [1987], defines *ototoxic* as "having a harmful effect on the organs or nerves concerned with hearing and balance.")

Dr. Paul Eric Hammerschlag, otological surgeon and otoneurologist at New York University Medical Center, New York City, a leading authority of ototoxicology, says, "I've had patients who have had hearing problems due to ototoxic drugs. Basically, the people were given drugs that were known to be potentially ototoxic, but I don't know at what dose level, whether it was above the therapeutic level or whether they had renal failure or other medical problems that would impair the excretion of this medication. Some of these people have been left with permanent hearing loss or permanent deficit in terms of vertigo. There are certain classes of drugs that have an affinity for the inner ear. If they are not successfully excreted by the kidneys or metabolized in the body, they are going to accumulate persistently to cause auditory or vestibular problems."

Dr. Joseph E. Hawkins, professor emeritus of physiological acoustics at the Kresge Hearing Research Institute at the University of Michigan Medical School in Ann Arbor and an early pioneer and investigator of ototoxic drugs, says, "Neomycin, the second of the important aminoglycosides, has proven to be ototoxic whether injected, taken orally, or used as a wash. Used as a wound irrigation, for example, it caused deafness in a number of cases. It is still used in ear drops and can cause considerable harm, particularly if the eardrum is perforated. It should be completely avoided."

Before her doctor prescribed diuretics, my friend Cynthia had mild hearing loss in one ear, the kind of loss that kept her from hearing announcements clearly when sitting at the rear of an auditorium and gave her some difficulty when she attended large functions where band music got in the way of her understanding group conversation. But her loss caused no hearing problem in most day-to-day activities. However, after a regimen of diuretics Cynthia had a dramatic hearing loss. No longer mild in just one ear, her loss became 50 percent bilaterally.

Dr. Linstrom says, "They are teaching about ototoxic drugs at the resident level, but they do not teach medical students about these drugs other than those for cancer chemotherapy."

Dr. Brummett agrees: "In residency otolaryngology programs residents are taught about drug-induced hearing loss but very little is taught in medical schools per se. I don't know why. In fact, the ear receives very little attention in medical schools. Many medical students have a very poor understanding even of the general anatomy of the auditory system. They certainly need to be made more aware of the effects of drugs on the auditory system."

Dr. Parmer recalls, "In medical school, which I attended many years ago, there was almost nothing taught that was relative to ototoxic medication."

Dr. Brummett says, "When I was a student, the main reason ototoxicity was mentioned was because of two drugs, the first being streptomycin, which had been out for a number of years and was known to damage the auditory system. At that time, all drugs that were called 'mycins' were colloquially called 'ototoxic mycins.' There was very little known about ototoxicity, and I wasn't taught anything more about it except that it occurred. The other drug with significant ototoxicity was aspirin.

"At the Oregon Health Sciences University at this time not a lot of emphasis is placed on ototoxicity. Medical students receive a little bit of information when they take pharmacology, and the reason is that I do some of that teaching. They also get some information about ototoxicity in public health courses, where I again talk to them. But there is no concentrated effort to teach ototoxicity."

My friend Cynthia says, "Isn't it unconscionable that I was put on large doses of diuretics! If I hadn't read an article about their potential for causing hearing loss, I might have continued taking those pills and become totally deaf. Fortunately, I found a doctor who got my blood pressure down with the 'Pritikin Approach.'"

Cynthia was determined to devote herself to gathering evidence about drug-induced deafness. She added her name to a list she was sure was miles long, a list of people who had become hearing disabled by drugs. We became partners, investigating menacing pills the hearing community and the already hearing-impaired community were being victimized by. On our daily walks we talked of little else besides drug-induced deafness.

Cynthia's house was a large, rambling colonial at the top of a village hill we climbed on our regular walks. As we approached it one day, she insisted I come inside. "I have something to show you about pills and hearing loss." These words got me to follow her enthusiastically into a large wood-paneled den where a desk was covered with pamphlets. She was really researching the subject of "sinful pills." There were letters and pamphlets from the National Institutes of Health (NIH). Page 16 of one pamphlet had been photocopied several times, and bold, angry strokes in red crayon underscored a paragraph about drug-induced hearing loss:

> *Drug-induced hearing loss.* Drugs as common as aspirin, the antibiotics streptomycin or neomycin, and certain of the water pills (diuretics) used to treat high blood pressure can damage the hair cells or other vital parts of the inner ear. Anyone who, while under medication, has a sudden change in hearing, or experiences dizziness or

ringing in the ears (tinnitus), or has other problems with hearing or balance should report the symptoms to a physician at once. Often changes in the prescription can eliminate the symptoms and prevent permanent damage to the ear. (National Institutes of Health, 1982)

"We really must distribute this to members of our SHHH group," said Cynthia. "Everyone has a right to know, and we have an obligation to enlighten them." Cynthia was eager for a campaign about sinful pills. The pamphlet only named aspirin, streptomycin, neomycin, and certain diuretics as offenders, but I got the feeling these were merely the tip of an iceberg.

Armed with page 16 of the NIH publication, I left Cynthia to begin my own long search for hearing-damaging drugs. From east coast to west coast, from north to south, I talked with doctors about pills that might have the potential to harm hearing. Some doctors told me about medications they believed should be avoided. Others talked about only a few suspect drugs. I pored over medical journals for concurrence about dangerous pills.

As I conferred with doctors and read journals, my list of dangerous pills grew, pills with such intimidating names that I needed intense concentration just to pronounce them properly. I needed to know which names were generic; which drugs were used commonly and which were reserved for life-threatening situations, where hearing loss does not have priority; and which drugs had viable substitutes and which did not.

I called on my pharmacist friend Ben, who worked at the pharmacy of one of the major hospitals on the North Shore of Long Island. He developed a list of his own for me. Some of his drugs were repeats of the drugs already on my list, but some were new additions. Ben also supplied me with an issue of the *Pharmacy Times* that discusses the ever-evolving body of evidence about drugs that can induce hearing disorders (Jinks, 1990).

Sitting in my office, a small room at the garden side of my house, writing about the psychological impact of hearing impairment on the impaired, as well as on their families and friends, and assembling my list of medications capable of damaging innocent ears, I would have the recurrent nightmarish thought that the public is poorly informed and insufficiently warned about drugs that can induce hearing disorders. Shouldn't these potential harmers be labeled as such when they are dispensed into a prescription container for the unsuspecting patient?

I decided to contact the Food and Drug Administration (FDA), although I had already determined from discussions with Ben that consumer packages of potentially ototoxic drugs are not labeled with warnings about the cochlear or vestibular damage they might produce, warnings about how extensively they could damage hair cells. There are 20,000 to 40,000 of these sensory fibers in the human ear; as they are destroyed, irreversible hearing loss results.

Sensory fiber damage can result from noise pollution, childhood diseases like scarlet fever, long bouts of high fever, and blows to the head. But the culprits I was after were the ototoxic pills ingested in all innocence: pills prescribed when viable substitutes were available; pills prescribed without proper monitoring; pills prescribed unknowledgeably, over too long a period of time; pills prescribed for non-life-threatening situations when other treatment methods might be available; and over-the-counter pills that, like aspirin, are commonly considered safe.

Searching for information about these harmful pills and lobbying to make it mandatory that pharmacists, filling prescriptions for potentially ototoxic medications, attach warning labels to alert the vulnerable hearing and hearing-impaired became my crusade. Warning labels are common enough:

MEDICATION SHOULD BE TAKEN WITH PLENTY OF WATER

MAY CAUSE DISCOLORATION OF URINE OR FECES

YOU SHOULD AVOID PROLONGED OR EXCESSIVE EXPOSURE TO
DIRECT AND/OR ARTIFICIAL SUNLIGHT WHILE TAKING THIS
MEDICATION

TAKE WITH FOOD OR MILK

DO NOT TAKE DAIRY PRODUCTS, ANTACIDS, OR IRON PREPA-
RATIONS WITHIN ONE HOUR OF THIS MEDICATION

MAY CAUSE DROWSINESS. USE CARE WHEN OPERATING A CAR
OR DANGEROUS MACHINERY

These are just a few examples of warning labels provided to pharmacists for application to prescription
drugs. *Not one* of all the labels provided to pharmacists
warns of potential ototoxicity.

Onward I went, to the FDA (the horse's mouth, so to
speak). Telephoning a government agency is not an easy
task for a person with severe hearing impairment. I made
many visits to my husband's office so he could come to
my assistance during my conversations with hasty and
indistinct voices from the Washington end of the line.
Twenty-five phone calls produced some amazing results.

One FDA staff member practically accused me of in-
vention: "Ototoxic! What's that? I've been with the
agency for twenty years, and I never heard the word." If
someone connected with the FDA for twenty years had
never heard the word *ototoxic*, how acquainted was the
public with the concept that medicines could cause hearing loss? On impulse, I checked several dictionaries. In
other than medical dictionaries, I could find *ototoxic* in
only *The Random House Dictionary, The American Heritage Dictionary* (third edition, 1992) and *Merriam-Web-
ster's Collegiate Dictionary* (tenth edition, 1993.)

Ototoxic does not appear in *Webster's Third New International Dictionary of the English Language* (unabridged, 1981).

Ototoxic does not appear in *Funk & Wagnall's New Standard Dictionary.*

Ototoxic does not appear in the *Oxford English Dictionary,* a supplement to the *Oxford English Dictionary* (1982).

Ototoxic does not appear in the *Oxford English Dictionary* (second edition, 1989 twenty volumes).

Ototoxic does not appear in *Grolier International Dictionary* (1981).

Ototoxic does not appear in *Third Barnhart Dictionary of New English* (1990).

Ototoxic does not appear in *Barnhart Dictionary of Etymology* (1988).

Ototoxic does not appear in *Chambers English Dictionary* (Cambridge University Press, 1988).

Ototoxic does not appear in *Longman Dictionary of the English Language* (new edition, 1991).

Ototoxic does not appear in *Oxford Encyclopedic English Dictionary* (1991).

Ototoxic does not appear in *The American Heritage Illustrated Encyclopedic Dictionary* (1987).

Some innocent conspiracy was keeping people with a full complement of healthy auditory hair cells from knowledge that could save their good hearing, and this same conspiracy was concealing knowledge from people with hearing impairment, knowledge that could help them preserve what hearing they had left, help them protect their remaining hair cells from further risk.

So it was back to my telephone calls to find a proper ally in the FDA. Persistence paid. Dr. F. Rosa, in the Division of Epidemiology and Surveillance (HFD-730), was not only knowledgeable but extremely interested in my project. The subject of our conversation, with my husband as a conduit, turned from the labeling of ototoxic drugs to the availability of lists of drugs that could cause deafness or hearing loss.

Dr. Rosa, representing public service at its best, renewed my faith in the enormous complex of government. He listened intently as I spoke about the need for a comprehensive drug list that would alert the hearing and the hearing-impaired communities to substances that could harm the ears. He told me, "Your analysis of this question should be of broad interest. We will look forward to seeing this when it is available."

I learned about the *Physicians' Desk Reference (PDR)*, a catalog of almost every known drug, and the *Drug Interactions and Side Effects Index* (keyed to the *PDR*), which contains lists of deafness-inducing and ototoxic drugs. Information in the *Physicians' Desk Reference* is supplied by drug companies. A phone call to the publisher uncovered the alarming fact that the *PDR*'s lists of deafness-inducing and ototoxic drugs only began appearing in the 1989 edition. On the positive side, these drugs are now listed in ready view for physicians who are willing to purchase a copy of the *Index*.

When I asked Dr. Linstrom about the ototoxic drugs listed in the *Index* and in other texts, he obliged me with a substantive discussion of drugs that can have harmful effects on the ears. For the better part of our 60-minute interview he spoke about the various classifications of drugs and the potential of each drug to harm hearing. It was as though he were quoting from a printed text, but he was not; this knowledge was printed on his brain. I left the interview with many, many pages for my comprehensive list of drugs that have the potential to damage the ears.

When I spoke with Dr. Parmer about the lists in the *Index*, he said, "There is so little available to the physician in the form of lists of drugs that are ototoxic. The lists in the *Drug Interactions and Side Effects Index* are almost useless because they are not complete. Apparently, someone goes through the *Physicians' Desk Reference,* looks into adverse reactions to drugs, and makes up a list.

"It is important to note that a very serious problem exists with the drug *gentamicin,* and gentamicin is not found in the *Drug Interactions and Side Effects Index.* Another point is that even this inadequate information is probably not available to most doctors who do not purchase the *Drug Interactions and Side Effects Index.* It then behooves the physician, when he prescribes a drug, to check the *Physicians' Desk Reference,* which is widely available. But even this process of checking for negative reactions regarding the eighth nerve, the auditory nerve, is not foolproof because the *Physicians' Desk Reference* does not in every case warn about potential ototoxicity."

Dr. Hawkins says, "The amount of time devoted to otolaryngology during the four years of medical school is really very small. The otolaryngologists who teach are more interested in basic principles—that is, how to examine ears—so they may never get around to strong warnings about ototoxicity. Of course, there should be some exposure to ototoxicity in pharmacology or in internal medicine. But sometimes these things fall between the cracks.

"Ototoxic medications are always described in the package insert with quite a full exposition of the side effects, uses, and dosages. Unfortunately, these are not always read by the prescriber. There's a lot of fine print there."

Dr. Berlin, Director of Louisiana State University Medical Center's Ear, Nose, and Throat Department's Kresge Hearing Research Laboratory of the South (New Orleans), says, "There's lengthy opportunity here for exposure to auditory physiology and ototoxic case analysis during the five years of residency. And warnings are almost always present in the physician's warning booklets in the drug package. To our knowledge, medical students and residents are being trained in this area, but whether they are being sufficiently trained to prevent any case of ototoxic drug mismanagement is hard to predict."

Dr. Hawkins told me about ototoxic drugs reaching the consumer without adequate testing: "I had been at Harvard working on auditory problems when Merck and Company asked me to work for them to investigate streptomycin. This was 1946, when the Mayo Clinic found that streptomycin was producing totally unexpected changes in vestibular function and in hearing (vestibular: balance, vertigo). The drug had not been adequately tested in animals before it was rushed to trial. Kanamycin was another drug rushed too quickly to trial. Neither was adequately tested before issued, and their ototoxic effects were first discovered in human patients."

Dr. Brummett told me that among the patients he had treated for hearing loss caused by ototoxic medication was an elderly woman who before receiving the medication had considered getting a hearing aid only because she had some minimal difficulty in group conversations. He said, "Subsequent to having her hearing tested, she was treated with an aminoglycoside antibiotic and a loop diuretic. This particular combination of drugs, if they are given in sufficient doses, can cause an immediate loss of hearing. This lady went from hearing that was almost so good she didn't have to wear a hearing aid to the point where a hearing aid wouldn't even help her. This happened within one month. Aminoglycosides and loop diuretics can cause an immediate and very dramatic permanent hearing loss."

Gathering information about ototoxic drugs and learning about the inadequacy of available lists and of drug testing, I thought about people with hearing impairment who have become dropouts because the hearing world intimidates them. How many could trace their problem to harmful pills? I thought too about the fortunate hearing people who stand at the precipice of hearing disorders, ready candidates to be pushed over the cliff by such pills. Sometimes I pictured those pills as tentacles waiting to pull in unsuspecting victims.

Forewarned may be forearmed, but how many in the hearing world even consider the possibility that an insidious pill can cause them to lose the vital sense that keeps them a part of normally functioning life—for without that precious sense of hearing there is surely no longer a normal life.

Everything changes when hearing impairment occurs. Not a second goes by without considering the events leading to that fateful day good hearing stopped. Like a stopped clock, the familiar routines of everyday life stagger and halt. Worse, die. Take early morning, for example. There is no alarm to ring you into your necessary pace. Searching for new ways to get yourself started at 7 AM, you lie awake for hours on end, or pray that your mental alarm will not fail. You haven't learned about the alarm clock that can shake you awake (see page 254).

The early morning radio news, accompanying an early morning shower and tooth-brushing drill, no longer exists. Scrap the radio! So how do you know road conditions when you get into your car? Take potluck and, often as not, end up on the one expressway the man in the helicopter has been urging the lucky ones with hearing to avoid. And this is only the beginning of your day!

The office intercom booms, and across your room flies babble. Lots of babble. The requisite morning office meeting is heated with controversy. There's kudos for those who can get their licks in, but you sit reticent, fearful of sounding foolish by repeating what an associate has just stated.

The morning is off to an inglorious start and all because of a little pill that could easily have been avoided with no risk to your good health. There were available substitutes, but you weren't in tune with this hazard in a country where there are miraculous medications, medications that can do so much good—and so much needless harm. You had no list of ototoxic drugs that you might have discussed with your physician.

Lunchtime is another hurdle. This hour of past pleasantries in a restaurant is now an assault to your ears. You understand nothing others at the table say. Better to eat alone, which you finally do, giving up a piece of business that could mean the difference between ordinary and top-drawer performance.

Your days and nights are governed by ears that no longer function for you, thanks—or no thanks—to harmful pills.

So how do I, a severely hearing-impaired nonmedical person, get the message across to my sisters and brothers in the hearing world? The "Beware the sinful pill" slogan is not sufficient. There ought to be a law. There ought to be a list.

I continue with my search through volumes, tomes, and texts, a search that takes me from Long Island's hospitals to the FDA; the New York Eye and Ear Hospital in New York City; New York University Medical Center in New York City; St. John's College of Pharmacy in Queens; the University of Michigan Medical Center in Ann Arbor; the House Ear Clinic in Los Angeles; Louisiana State University Medical Center in New Orleans; Oregon Health Sciences University School of Medicine in Portland; and other facilities that can help me develop a comprehensive list of deafness-inducing and ototoxic drugs.

Where does responsibility for wider knowledge about ototoxic drugs begin? Why is this aspect of medicine so neglected? Dr. Parmer says, "In reference to the consideration given to ototoxic medications in today's medical schools: there is not too much taught, although the ear, nose, and throat departments and the courses in pharmacology do alert future physicians to the fact that drugs can cause hearing loss and vestibular problems.

"The brochure that comes with drugs is another source of information. However, it is a false sense of security if one believes doctors get information from these brochures, since the doctor rarely sees the brochure with the drug—certainly not with those drugs that are administered intravenously or in the hospital setting. The doctor has nothing to do with the administration of the drug other than to prescribe the proper dose and follow the blood levels. He will not be exposed to the brochure which comes with the container of the drug to be administered to the patient."

Dr. Linstrom says, "I went to school in Canada, where we were taught about ototoxic drugs in medical school. At New York Eye and Ear Hospital, I receive the *Medical Letter* every two weeks, which reports about new drugs, including their known toxicities. But I believe most doctors limit themselves to approximately thirty drugs that they know very well.

"Any new drug that is going to be introduced in the hospital must go before the committee to review known adverse side effects. But some medications that we have to use in extremis will cause hearing loss.

"I think the best thing would be for the FDA to make available an easily understandable fact sheet [about ototoxicity], particularly for medications that are taken by a patient for an entire lifetime."

When I talked with Dr. Brummett, he returned to the question of testing new drugs: "I give a course on drug-induced hearing loss at the American Academy of Otolaryngology. I've done it for the past twelve years and will again this fall. One of the problems is that when new drugs are developed there are no requirements that these drugs be tested for potential ototoxicity before they are put into human beings.

"When new chemicals that may have an effect on the

auditory system are being developed, that effect is first discovered in man. Then it is confirmed in laboratory animals. I know of no exceptions to this rule. You might argue that this is not true for 'me too' drugs. For example, after the prototype loop diuretic, ethacrynic acid, was found to be ototoxic in human beings, laboratory tests were done with other loop diuretics before they were dispensed to man.

"After streptomycin was found to be ototoxic, other aminoglycoside antibiotics that were developed were tested in laboratory animals. But if you take a brand new drug, a new chemical, it is not tested for ototoxicity before it is released.

"I was in touch with the FDA about the need for a testing program for new drugs, and they did send me a proposal, which I reviewed and sent back to them. But I never heard anything more about it. It seems to me that if the FDA required new drugs to be tested for ototoxicity in laboratory animals, this would focus attention on the problem. This is something that needs to be paid attention to."

When I arrived at the New York University Medical Center in New York City to interview Dr. Paul Eric Hammerschlag, he had a thin book waiting for me on his desk: *Handbook of Ototoxicity,* by Dr. Julian J. Miller (1985), principal scientific officer at the Wessex Regional Health Authority, Winchester, England. This book is one of the most helpful texts I have come across. It is filled with documented evidence of toxicity for all the drugs it cites as potentially ototoxic.

Reading through Dr. Miller's book, I came across two pages about the antibiotic ampicillin. Ampicillin was already on my list of suspected offenders. It is listed as ototoxic in *Otolaryngology,* edited by Gerald M. English (1983), and in the chapter on ototoxicity in *Diseases of the Ear* (Stringer, Meyerhoff, & Wright, 1991). However, numerous physicians I talked with freely prescribed ampicillin and were skeptical about the listing of it as ototoxic. They asked for evidence. In his *Handbook of Ototoxicity,* Julian Miller (1985) devotes two pages (pp. 97–98) to case studies of hearing loss following ampicillin treatment.

My main or first listing singles out medications that fall into the category of drugs generally accepted as dangerous. My second list identifies medications and other substances that are controversial. The third list includes substances that have ototoxic consequences in rare cases (frequently, studies have found, these substances have reversible ototoxic effects, but people with already damaged ears, ears that may be predisposed to harm from relatively safe or mildly ototoxic medications, may want to avoid them).

In developing my lists it was not my purpose to warn people with life-threatening illness that they had better protect their ears. It is my crusade to protect people with non-life-threatening illnesses—the "sinful pill" victim—who could have been treated satisfactorily with a benign substitute.

My friend Cynthia, one of the 17 million people with sensorineural hearing loss, gives doctors no out for lack of knowledge about the pills that separated her from the hearing world, no out for condemning her to the isolation that comes with "the territory." No Pollyanna complex forgives them for her loss. Nothing can make it better.

Suffering the consequences of harmful pills, Cynthia thinks each day has value only if I succeed in adding to my list—which may be the only comprehensive one—of ototoxic drugs. I remind Cynthia that I am not a physician, that my knowledge of the drugs about which I am gathering information is far from profound. All I really am is a listener and a lister. (Fortunate that two of Long Island's most prestigious hospitals are a stone's throw from my home, I listen and I list.)

These hospitals have formulary committees that review and recommend drugs for approved use at the hospital. I had hoped that the chairperson of the committee at the first hospital I telephoned would peruse my growing list of ototoxic drugs and discuss with me the best way for patients to be spared hearing loss produced by pills that could adversely affect sensory hair cells. But he declined to meet with me, saying that he felt inadequate and uncomfortable with the subject of ototoxic medicines. The library at this first hospital did not stock what many doctors consider a basic text, namely, *The Drug Interactions and Side Effects Index.*

I had better luck at the second hospital, where Dr. Leo Parmer is chairperson of the formulary committee. Better luck too with the library at this second hospital. The librarian at Long Island Jewish Medical Center directed me to the library copy of *Meyler's Side Effects of Drugs* (Dukes, 1988). This encyclopedia contains a short list (eight items to be exact) of deafness-inducing drugs. The library also has the current edition of *Drug Interactions and Side Effects Index.* In addition, it has *Textbook of Adverse Drug Reactions* (third edition), edited by D. M. Davies, a consulting physician and editor of the *Adverse Drug Reaction Bulletin;* this text also contains a short list (fifteen items) of major ototoxic drugs, which are analyzed for their propensity to cause degeneration of the sensory hair cells, that is, hearing loss.

From the helpful librarian at Long Island Jewish Medical Center I went to the helpful man who chairs the formulary committee. Dr. Parmer was admirably candid in admitting that he had previously not been deeply involved with ototoxic drugs and had not discussed ototoxicity in his newsletters. However, he was extremely interested in the subject and in my project and said he would deal with ototoxic drugs in future newsletters.

Some of the physicians I talked with did not encourage my search for harmful pills. The doctor at the Manhattan Eye and Ear Hospital was concerned that my thrust might be antidoctor. Dr. Hammerschlag of the New York University Medical Center, who supplied me with the very helpful text on ototoxicity by Julian Miller (1985), assured me that my list "will be helpful to both the physician and the patient" at the same time that he urged caution: "If your list contains drugs that are questionably ototoxic, it won't be authoritative. The questionably ototoxic drugs can undermine the validity of the entire list."

I do not take these concerns and warnings lightly, and hasten to assure all those who question my crusade to shine a beacon of light on the potential hazards to the human ear that I am not antidoctor and neither is my crusade. On the contrary, my search for and disclosure of potentially ototoxic drugs is a crusade the medical community might well have undertaken itself. But physicians are trapped in a Catch-22 situation. Doctors want to know which drugs may be ototoxic. They want to protect the hearing of patients who are not hearing impaired, and they do not want to worsen the hearing of those patients who already have hearing loss. Yet their concerns about malpractice and their mountains of paperwork make them most unlikely to report hearing loss or deafness resulting from medications they have prescribed. Without this reporting, the FDA lacks evidence about the magnitude of damage pills and other medications are inflicting on the public and is therefore unable to issue warnings to doctors.

Dr. Parmer explained the problem: When the procedure for reporting adverse drug reactions at his hospital was the sole responsibility of doctors, two or three cases were reported monthly. When the procedure was changed, giving the hospital pharmacologists responsibility for reading patients' charts, ten to fifteen cases were reported each month. The hospital, in making this change, was surely not antidoctor; it simply recognized, as I do, the many problems inherent in having physicians report adverse reactions to the medications they have prescribed.

To address the possibility that my list contains drugs that may be questionably ototoxic, I must state that I am simply a listener and a compiler. I have talked with doctors across the country and researched more than twenty-five sources for potentially ototoxic pills and other medications and I merely present my compilation for examination by those more qualified than I to judge dangers, risks, and benefits. Surely, in life-threatening circumstances, the scale weighs in favor of the benefit. In other circumstances, there may be substitutes and alternatives for the potentially ototoxic drug.

I present my compilation so that consumers will have the opportunity to explore the risks and benefits for themselves. My comprehensive list of potentially ototoxic medications should be a welcome service to the medical community (by which I mean doctors other than otolaryngologists, otorhinolaryngologists, and otologists). Ear specialists are usually well educated in medicines that can harm the hearing; but it is all the other doctors, who are more likely to prescribe medications that may be potentially ototoxic, who should have a comprehensive list of potentially ototoxic drugs readily available.

In the preferred texts of physicians at the nation's most renowned hospitals and of the scientists at the Kresge hearing centers, I continue to search for references to medications and substances various physicians have suggested for my lists. I list and I worry that all the ingesting of little pills is like Russian roulette. Which, indeed, of the thousands and thousands of pills on the market can blow away delicate hair cells in a healthy ear? Which can further harm the already damaged ear, the ear with a predisposition to harm from even mildly ototoxic medication? In the absence of a comprehensive list, in the absence of conclusive warnings from the FDA, how do physicians protect their patients' hearing?

Dr. Linstrom says, "In using a potentially ototoxic drug, monitoring it is incumbent. It becomes my responsibility to monitor for side effects."

Dr. Parmer says, "Even when physicians are warned about possible ototoxic problems associated with new drugs, it is extremely difficult for the physician to know when the drugs produce ototoxic results. When the drug first comes on the medical market, blood levels for these drugs are not done routinely, so there may be cases of deafness produced by these drugs. In fact, there are cases where a wound was irrigated with an aminoglycoside such as neomycin and a sufficient amount of this drug was absorbed. Hearing loss followed.

"There is also the problem with senior citizens, who probably already have minor hearing problems. The effect of these drugs on people who already have a hearing problem becomes additive.

"One of the most important considerations in using these drugs is to determine how well the kidneys function. The kidneys are the major route for the excretion of some drugs. If the kidneys do not work properly, the blood level rises rapidly and deafness can ensue.

"There are also other risks involved with aminoglycoside drugs. Prolonged use, even despite proper blood levels, could result in ototoxicity. Repeated use—or, as it is called medically, 'sequential use'—could do the same.

"The question arises as to how practicing physicians can avoid damaging the eighth nerve of their patients."

On the subject of monitoring ototoxic drugs Dr. Brummett says, "Monitoring requires sophisticated audiometric testing by someone professionally trained, like an audiologist. These people are not necessarily available in all hospitals. The other problem is that you need patients who are reasonably alert to cooperate in having their hearing tested.

"Having hearing tested can be exhausting for a hospital patient. It can also be quite uncomfortable. Physicians don't have an easy way to follow hospital patients to whom they are giving ototoxic drugs.

"We desperately need a simple test, for monitoring on a daily basis, to find out if there is change in the auditory function. This is not possible today. We are, however, working at developing such a device, which will heighten awareness about people who are given potentially ototoxic drugs.

"What we're working on is a pen-size object which the physician will be able to hold up to the patient's ear to monitor on a daily basis to see whether there has been any change in the auditory function."

When I talked with Dr. Robert Mangione, R.Ph., M.S., the assistant dean of pharmacy student affairs and clinical professor of pharmacy at St. John's University in Queens, New York, he discussed the monitoring role of the pharmacist in a hospital setting: "Pharmacists in a hospital setting should receive reports of patients who develop hearing loss while on medication. They are appropriately educated and scientifically trained to be actively involved in this area. It is an aspect of pharmacy practice the profession would embrace.

"Pharmacists in the hospital setting can look for a relationship between the dose and the blood serum level. They can be actively involved in helping prevent adverse effects.

"And the patient has a right to know if a drug is considered potentially ototoxic. There should be cooperation among all the health professionals—the physician, the pharmacist, and the nurse—to weigh the risk against the benefit.

"In the community setting it is not as easy as in the hospital setting. People go to more than one pharmacy, and they may go to more than one doctor. There may be no one source with knowledge of the person's entire medical history, no one source to say to the consumer of a potentially ototoxic drug, 'Watch out for this. Be sure to be monitored when taking this.'

"If people were aware of potentially ototoxic medications, they could look into therapeutic alternatives. This is a challenge in ambulatory situations. So it is important that people be educated about medications. If they received a list of potentially ototoxic drugs with a first hearing aid, it would be a step in the direction of better awareness."

About monitoring, Dr. Parmer says, "One of the major problems with drugs that induce eighth-nerve damage is the process of monitoring these drugs. Unless a doctor tests his patients with audiometric tests constantly as the patient uses an ototoxic drug, the doctor will not know what he is dealing with. Constant audiometric testing is a very expensive and impractical approach. So the question is, How does the doctor find out about ototoxicity in drugs he is prescribing?"

Dr. Parmer continues: "The FDA requests, but does not require, that doctors send in a form called an Adverse Drug Reaction when they run into a problem—a hearing problem or other kind of problem. Unfortunately, doctors rarely fill out these forms for every ill effect they see. If the side effect has already been written up in the literature, the doctor will say to himself, 'Why should I bother notifying the FDA? They already know about this problem.'

"However, if there was mandatory reporting of every kind of drug reaction, the FDA would be made aware of problems long before they now become aware of the extent of the problem."

Dr. Hammerschlag adds, "Mandatory reporting to the FDA could be helpful so it can ascertain the extent of hearing loss caused by a drug. We're acquainted with the odd case here and there. Yet I'm not acquainted with an excessive number of patients or a large volume of cases of ototoxicity, which may suggest that the incidence of ototoxic side effects is low. I'm not being cavalier. If a drug has an adverse effect on one person when some other medication could have been given, that is one person too many. Mandatory reporting would be helpful so the FDA could send out advisory newsletters confirming which drugs are ototoxic. Unfortunately, physicians are already overwhelmed by paperwork, so it is difficult to anticipate more mandatory reporting to the FDA."

Dr. Hawkins says, "The medical profession tries, but they don't always succeed. Reports to the FDA about adverse effects should be encouraged, but I don't know whether making this reporting mandatory would help. Physicians' enormous amounts of paperwork would still tend to make them neglect reporting."

Without adequate reporting to the FDA, there is inadequate reporting from the FDA back to physicians about drugs that have produced hearing loss. This makes it more urgent for patients to be monitored when they are on medication that may possibly harm their hearing.

Dr. Hawkins says, "We have asked physicians to give close attention to patients' complaints about tinnitus [ringing in the ear], dizziness, vertigo, anything that might arouse suspicion about ototoxicity. I don't think it's possible to expect every patient to be given an audiogram or a vestibular workup every day or every week. One has to depend very largely on the patients' own reports.

"Patients should be made aware that they are getting a potentially ototoxic drug and should be sure to note if there is any sign of auditory or vestibular disturbance. With some patients this is not possible—infants, people who are very sick or senile. Pediatricians and other physicians must be very careful about drugs they choose. Although sometimes the choice may not be very wide. And I think there is a tendency for doctors to choose the latest drug, which may not always be the safest."

My friend Cynthia is exasperated when I tell her what many of our nation's leading authorities on ototoxicity say about monitoring. "It comes down to this," Cynthia complains. "People with hearing impairment had better take charge of their own problem. People with auditory systems predisposed to harm from suspect medication had better know which medications to avoid, when the avoiding is possible. When the avoiding is impossible, we'd better be sure we're properly monitored."

Like Cynthia, Dr. Parmer becomes my partner in poring over books and articles with references to potentially ototoxic drugs. He says, "Another problem with the lists in the *Drug Interactions and Side Effects Index* and some of the other texts is that the name of the drug is frequently the trade name and not the generic name. They should list both. A doctor may not be familiar with the trade name and therefore when prescribing a generic drug, even looking at these texts, may not realize that that drug may be ototoxic.

"Changes can be made in the practice of medicine in order to avoid the danger of ototoxicity. When drugs of different varieties are prescribed over a period of many years, each of these drugs may perhaps have a minor effect, but all together they may be additive in doing eighth-nerve damage. In other words, a patient may find, or contend, that he or she has a hearing loss. But it is impossible to look back, the way medicine is practiced today, to determine whether this is a naturally occurring or aging process or whether doctors over the years have prescribed drugs that may have produced small amounts of damage that are additive.

"The solution to this problem is rather complicated but not unattainable. Most doctors keep records of their patients. When a new patient comes in, they take a history. There is always a place in the history for allergies. Most doctors will take a complete history of which drugs the patient is allergic to. It is just as important to take a listing of all drugs the patient has taken over the years. Keep these in a separate part of the history form. When the doctor prescribes a drug he knows may be ototoxic, he will record the fact. He now has a means of following all possible administration of ototoxic drugs."

In *Ototoxicity in Infant and Fetus: Childhood Deafness* (1977), Dr. Hawkins discusses the problem of the youngest members of our society who are without the precious sense of hearing. Dr. Hawkins explains that the immature renal system in premature babies puts their auditory systems at extreme risk from aminoglycoside medications. He also explains that the auditory systems of the pregnant mother and her fetus are at considerable risk when the mother uses ototoxic diuretics.

Scientists like Dr. Hawkins and our country's leading physicians provided the foundation for this chapter on ototoxicity. I am not a physician and make no claim to knowing how the hearing and the hearing-impaired should deal with their bodies when it comes to pills prescribed by their physicians. I am saying only that patients deserve the opportunity to understand the possible side effects of the pills being prescribed for their various ailments. They deserve the opportunity to question risk factors, the opportunity to select between potential danger and viable nontoxic substitutes, the opportunity to have in hand a comprehensive ototoxic drug list on which to base a discussion of the treatment proposed by their doctor.

The list I am working with keeps growing because I know that every day innocent ears are falling victim to drugs that can damage their hearing. A mother should know if her child is taking a pill that can cause an irreversible hearing disorder. People who still possess their good hearing should be aware that they can become residents of the world of the 28 million hearing-disabled because a little pill can lead them there. The mildly, the moderately, and the severely hearing-disabled deserve to be alerted to the fact that their insufficient hearing can be further damaged if they swallow certain little pills.

Chapter 12

Deafening Medications

There are many contributors to hearing loss, including sickness, birth complications, blows to the head, genetic disorders. These may be beyond the control of the families of the afflicted or the afflicted themselves. There are, however, certain contributors that can be controlled or eliminated by knowledgeable family members or the potential victim. Caution about medicines can save hearing. This chapter deals with ototoxic (harmful to ears) medications.

Physicians and Scientists

Investigating medications and other substances that may be responsible for hearing loss, I talked with many, many physicians, scientists, ototoxicologists, and pharmacists. The following experts were interviewed at length for Chapters 10, 11, and 12.

CHARLES I. BERLIN, Ph.D., Director of Louisiana State University Medical Center's Ear, Nose, and Throat Department's Kresge Hearing Research Laboratory of the South (New Orleans); Clinical Professor, Department of Psychology, University of New Orleans, New Orleans, Louisiana; and Director, Audiology Services, Department of Otolaryngology, Louisiana State University Medical Center. Dr. Berlin was awarded First Place for Scientific Merit by the American Speech and Hearing Association and has received the Award for Distinguished Services, American Academy of Ophthalmology and Otolaryngology.

ROBERT E. BRUMMETT, Ph.D., Professor of Otolaryngology and Pharmacology, Oregon Hearing Research Center, Oregon Health Sciences University, Portland, Oregon. His study is the effect of drugs on the auditory system. Dr. Brummett, perhaps our country's leading ototoxicologist, was on the advisory board for the *Handbook of Ototoxicity* (Miller, 1985).

PAUL ERIC HAMMERSCHLAG, M.D., F.A.C.S., Otological Surgeon and Otoneurologist at the New York University Medical Center, New York City. Dr. Hammerschlag is a leading authority on ototoxicology.

JOSEPH E. HAWKINS, Ph.D., D. Sc., Professor Emeritus of Physiological Acoustics at Kresge Hearing Research Institute, Department of Otorhinolaryngology, University of Michigan Medical School, Ann Arbor, Michigan. A pioneer investigator of ototoxic drugs and recipient of an Alexander von Humboldt Award for Senior U.S. Scientists, Dr. Hawkins was in Germany from June through December 1991 to research the history of otology. Dr. Hawkins, a former Rhodes Scholar, is also Distinguished Visiting Professor of Biology at Baylor University in Waco, Texas.

CHRISTOPHER J. LINSTROM, M.D., Fellow of the Royal College of Surgeons, Canada; Fellow of the American Academy of Otolaryngology/Head and Neck Surgery; Assistant Director of Otology, the New York Eye and Ear Infirmary, New York City; Assistant Professor of Otolaryngology, the New York Medical College; State Senatorial Scholarship, University of Maryland; Royal Society for the Advancement of Learning, McGill University; Friends of McGill Scholarship.

ROBERT A. MANGIONE, R.Ph., M.S., Assistant Dean, Pharmacy Student Affairs and Clinical Professor of Pharmacy at St. John's University, Queens, New York.

LEO G. PARMER, M.D., Ph.D., Pharmacology, Columbia University; M.D., Columbia University College of Physicians and Surgeons. Dr. Parmer was with the Food and Drug Administration for eight years, part of the time as Deputy Medical Director. For the past 35 years he has been Chairperson of the Pharmacy and Therapeutics Committee at Long Island Jewish Medical Center, Queens, New York, which includes Schneider Children's Hospital and Hillside Hospital. Dr. Parmer is the medical consultant to the St. John's University Drug Information Service, a member of the Institutional Review Board of St. John's University, and Emeritus Assistant Professor of Clinical Medicine at Stony Brook Medical School.

Researching ototoxic substances, I consulted frequently with:

ELLIOTT C. GREENFIELD, M.D., Diplomate, American Board of Otolaryngology and Assistant Clinical Professor, Cornell University Medical College, FACS FALROF FAOHNS.

B<small>ENJAMIN</small> Z<small>ELDIN</small>, Ph.G, B.Sc. in Pharmacy.

And others too numerous to name.

Potentially Ototoxic Medications and Substances

To develop lists of potentially ototoxic drugs and substances, I consulted with numerous doctors, scientists, and pharmacists. Over the course of a year, Dr. Leo Parmer worked with me to organize my three lists. Together we studied the texts and journals recommended by the physicians and scientists I interviewed. We also studied texts and journals recommended by hospital librarians. It is our hope that consumers and physicians may find the reference section of this book useful for their own investigation of the ototoxicity of the drugs and substances included in the three lists.

When examining the following lists of substances, it is essential to consider the risk—benefit factor; when a life-threatening disease is involved, hearing is *not* of prime importance.

The innumerable drugs and substances that may have adverse side effects on the vestibular system—that is, that may cause balance problems, vertigo, or dizziness—are *not* included in these lists. The three lists are concerned with hearing: sensorineural loss or tinnitus (ringing in the ear). Drugs that may produce tinnitus are of particular concern because tinnitus is frequently a precursor of hearing loss.

Some studies show that tinnitus or deafness can be caused by certain birth control medications. However, formulas are constantly changing, and these hearing problems may have resulted from early formulas. For this reason birth control pills are not included in the lists.

LIST 1. The Most Dangerous Medications and Substances Most Physicians and Scientists Consider Ototoxic

Generic Name	*Trade Name*
Acetylsalicylic acid (aspirin)	
(The hearing loss and tinnitus caused by aspirin are usually reversible.)	
Amikacin	Amikin
Amphotericin B	Fungizone
Bumetanide	Bumex
Capreomycin	Capastat
Carboplatin	Paraplatin
Chloroquine	Aralen
Cisplatin	Platinol
Ethacrynic acid	Edecrin
Furosemide	Lasix
Gentamicin	Garamycin
Hydroxychloroquine	Plaquenil
Kanamycin	Kantrex
Neomycin	Neomycin Sulfate Tablets Neosporin Irrigant, et al.
Salicylates/Methyl Salicylate/Oil of Wintergreen	Ben Gay (contains Methyl Salicylate 15%)
Streptomycin (only available from the U.S. Center for Disease Control for certain cases of tuberculosis)	
Tobramycin sulfate	Nebcin
Vancomycin	Vancocin
Viomycin	Viocin

LIST 2. Controversial Medications and Substances Many Physicians and Scientists Consider Potentially Ototoxic

Generic Name	*Trade Name*
Adrenacorticotropic hormone (ACTH)	Acthar
Auronofin (gold)	Ridaura
Betaxolol	Kerlone
Bleomycin	Blenoxane
Bromocriptine	Parlodel
Chloramphenicol	Chloromycetin
Erythromycin	ERYC, E-Mycin
Ibuprofen	Motrin, Advil et al.
Imipramine	Tofranil
Indomethacin	Indocin
Lead	
Mechlorethamine hydrochloride (Nitrogen Mustard)	Mustargen
Methyclothiazide	Aquatensen, Enduron
Misoprostol	Cytotec
Quinidine	Quinaglute, Quinadex
Quinine sulfate	Quinamm Tablets
Tolmetin	Tolectin

LIST 3. Medications and Substances That in Rare Cases May Be Ototoxic. (Ototoxicity of medications and substances on this list may be considered reversible. People with predisposition may want to avoid these suspects if substitutes are available.)

Generic Name	*Trade Name*
Acetazolamide	Diamox
Alcohol	
Atropine sulfate	
Ampicillin	Polycillin, Omnipen, et al.
Chlordiazepoxide	Librium

Chlorhexidine gluconate skin cleanser	Hibiclens Antimicrobial, Phisohex
Chloroform	
Chlorpheniramine maleate	Chlor-Trimeton, et al.
Clemastine fumarate	Tavist
Chlomipramine hydro-chloride	Anafranil
Dexchlorpheniramine	Polaramine
Dyclonine hydrochloride	Dyclone
Fluorouracil	Fluorouracil
Gallium nitrate	Ganite
Indapamide	Lozol
Iodine	Iodoform
Isoniazid	INH
Mannitol	Mannitol
Medroxyprogesterone ace-tate	Depo-Provera
Mefenamic acid	Ponstel
Mercury	
Methenamine mandelate	Mandelamine
Methyl alcohol	
Minocycline hydrochlo-ride	Minocin
Nalidixic acid	NegGram
Naproxen	Anaprox, Naprosyn
Phenylbutazone	Butazolidin
Phenytoin	Dilantin
Pilocarpine	Pilocar, Pilostat
Sulindac	Clinoril
Toluene (an industrial substance)	
Trichloroethylene (an in-dustrial substance)	

To add to these lists of potentially otototoxic medications and substances, Dr. Brummett sent me the following generic list. For the convenience of readers who may

not be acquainted with the generic names, I have added
trade names.

Generic Name	Trade Name
Amoxicillin	Amoxil
Azithromycin	Zithromax
Cinoxacin	Cinobac
Ciprofloxacin	Cipro
Clarithromycin	Biaxin
Diclofenac	Voltaren
Diflunisal	Dolobid
Fenoprofen	Nalfon
Griseofulvin	Fulvicin
Ketoprofen	Orudis
Meclofenamate	Meclofenamate
Netilmicin	Netromycin
Norfloxacin	Noroxin
Piroxicam	Feldene
Valproic Acid	Depakene

Postscript on Pills

I conclude a final session with Dr. Parmer, a session
devoted to organizing lists of dangerous medicines and
other substances. My three lists are put to bed, and my
husband says it is time I put myself to bed as well.

All the shuttling back and forth, from typewriter to
computer to hundreds of pages that need collating, has
made its mark on my index finger. I toss and turn in bed,
my finger throbbing from paper cuts. Out of bed I creep,
careful not to disturb my husband, who has been patient
enough with my erratic hours. Sorting through tubes in
the medicine cabinet, I feel a surge of pride that I am so
qualified to check the ingredients of the medication I will
be applying to a hurt finger. My lists will serve me well.

I seize a tube of medication recently prescribed for a skin irritation my husband had. Many months of delving into dangerous chemicals have taught me that it is more than pills than can harm the hearing. Liquids, injections, topically applied creams, cleaning fluids, and countless preparations threaten all of us, the hearing and the hearing impaired. I will check carefully before I put a speck of cream on my throbbing finger. Slapped on the part of the tube where ingredient information is printed is the druggist's label, with recommendations about using the cream. The description of the chemical contents is obscured, and there is no removing the druggist's overpasted label without removing all the print beneath it.

So, what's a person to do? My clever lists will not avail me in the least. Finger throbbing, I want to laugh, but I am filled with pain and fury.

Chapter 13

Update on Deafening Medications

When the hardcover edition of *When The Hearing Gets Hard* was published, booksellers were shocked when they thumbed through the pages of ototoxic (toxic to ears) medications. Most had never heard that word before.

In my mail came sad letters from men and women in all parts of our country describing hearing loss they attributed to medications. Some had had life-threatening illnesses but the vast majority had had no need for these potentially deafening drugs. They could have used benign alternative medications.

When I went on promotional tours, I met people who were angry that they were never warned that medications their doctors prescribed could make them deaf.

On one tour I met Bernice Roginski. Bernice and her husband lived on a farm in Salem Township, Michigan. Their children all adults, Bernice and her husband honeymooned weekends on their farm and, in nearby South Lyon, they knuckled down to business—selling real estate. Bernice loved her farm kitchen. Through closed windows she could hear the sounds of the country—bird music, breezes whistling among tree branches, the soft sighs of summer, the crispness of autumn—her hearing was that keen.

Bernice was baking a ham and tending a farm-size pot of soup boiling on her stove. She bent over to open the oven door and the soup pot rocked and flew, toppling steaming liquid on Bernice's back. In Ann Arbor's University of Michigan Hospital she was rushed to the care of a doctor from the burn unit. Nurses applied a prescribed salve to her back, all the while chatting with her about her accident.

A week after the salve applications began, the doctor asked Bernice if she was hard of hearing. Bernice said, "No, why do you ask?" The doctor said, "Because you keep asking me to repeat."

The nurses and Bernice's husband also noticed that her hearing was failing but the doctor did not have the applications of salve discontinued.

From her hospital bed Bernice kept in touch with her office. Then, one day she couldn't, not efficiently.

Bernice, an intelligent, well-educated woman, wondered if the salve being applied to her back could be the culprit. The nurses also fingered the salve. They talked with the doctor who dismissed the salve as a cause for the change in Bernice's hearing and ordered the nurses to continue its application. In four months Bernice's ears were irreversibly damaged. She could hear no more.

For all intents and purposes the person Bernice had been was gone. To people with healthy hearing, this may seem a harsh appraisal. But people who hear no more will testify that losing the precious sense of hearing haunts every aspect of life.

When I spoke to Bernice's lawyer he said, "The attendant physician should have known the ototoxicity of the drug (Neomycin). When Bernice started to demonstrate the loss of hearing, the administration of that drug should have been terminated."

A lawsuit was settled in Bernice's favor, but can any settlement compensate for the hearing of a widow with a business to run? I met Bernice twelve years after her doctor ordered the application of Neomycin that made her deaf. Her anger at the doctor and the hospital probably softened after twelve years of bereavement, but still she keeps reliving the time she lay on her stomach while nurses salved her back until she could hear no more. Those sterile walls will always close her in.

Joseph Tripi goes for therapy to the Hearing Center at The Long Island Jewish Medical Center in Queens, New York. When I interviewed him in October 1994 he told me about his hearing disorder which he first noticed in 1990. He had been taking Neomycin orally for two and a half years. In 1987 he had hepatitis and was hospitalized for 17 days. His medication in the hospital included Spironolactone, Cephulac (Lactulose) and Furosemide (Lasix). When he left the hospital, Neomycin tablets were added to his battery of medications. Within two months he noticed a hearing problem which he discussed with his doctor, who dismissed Neomycin as a cause. By 1991 he was totally deaf. An eminent otologist at New York University Hospital told him Neomycin could certainly have caused his deafness. His doctor disagreed and told him he needed to continue taking Neomycin to help him get "back to himself." Joseph Tripi believed that the doctor at NYU was correct and stopped taking Neomycin. There has been no adverse change in his condition since he went off the Neomycin.

Before his Neomycin experience Joseph Tripi was a land developer and a general contractor. He told me, "I worked in Texas, Florida, New York, New Jersey, Pennsylvania. I made a very good living. I never had a hearing problem. My wife Martha and I have been married thirty-nine years. We have three children and none of them have hearing problems. No one in my family has ever had hearing problems. Before that medication in the hospital and after I was out of the hospital, my hearing was absolutely normal. Now my hearing loss is profound. I am totally deaf. When they put me on the diuretic Furosemide or Lasix in the hospital and continued it and added Neomycin when I got out of the hospital, they should have warned me that those medications could cause hearing loss. I didn't get a word of warning. When I told the gastroenterologist who prescribed Neomycin and Lasix that I thought those medicines were making me lose my hearing, he said 'Don't worry about it. None of my patients ever got deaf from those medications so just continue taking the Neomycin.'

"The interesting thing is my wife took our poodle to a vet and mentioned my hearing problem and that I was on Neomycin. The vet told her, 'We used to use Neomycin on puppies and dogs but stopped when we found out it was making them deaf.'

"My deafness has changed my whole life. I had to close my business. I couldn't communicate and I would get frustrated and people I was dealing with would get frustrated trying to talk to me.

"I had to give up old friends because I was embarrassed. Some of them wanted to visit but I discouraged that because I couldn't hear. I'm a gregarious person, it's part of my life to be social, but I couldn't socialize anymore. I talk to my dog and my family. That's it! My brother lives in Florida and I can't even talk to him. My wife talks to him. I tried hearing aids. Four of them in fact. But none did me any good. I'm still paying for the last set of hearing aids I purchased. I'm learning to lipread.

"I get very angry because no doctor warned me I could become deaf from these medicines. What makes me so angry is that doctors don't all do their homework. They don't all know that medicines can make a person deaf.

Now I tell everyone 'Be careful if you go to a hospital. Be careful about medications. Don't use anything until you really look into the damage it can do to you. Maybe you have to take it but maybe you don't have to take it. Maybe you can take some other medicine that won't make you deaf.' "

Joseph Tripi's wife Martha is angry not only because the doctor who prescribed the Neomycin did not warn about its potential ototoxic effect but because there was no warning on the package.

Joseph Tripi's deafness made it impossible for him to continue functioning within the business world. Bernice Roginski's ability to function within her business world was so remarkable and probably so rare that the Detroit Free Press did a feature story about her in October 1993.

If the story of Bernice Roginski's experience with topical application of Neomycin had been well known within the medical community, the ears of a woman in Texas might have been saved.

Darrell Keith Esq. relates the case of his client Alberta Wells:

"At the time Alberta Wells went into the hospital she was a retired widow in her early to mid-sixties. She had developed a problem over her shoulder area, a pocket of infection. She was taken into surgery for the purpose of exploring that area. The surgeon determined that there was a large infection and he proceeded to clean the area. Then he irrigated the area with a solution that contained the antibiotic Neomycin.

"The surgeon was a thoracic and cardiovascular surgeon. He believed antibiotic irrigation therapy was useful and effective in treating surgical wounds in the chest or the thoracic area. He used Neomycin as a surgical irrigant because it had been used for that purpose for many years.

"In the litigation, it was our position that in their labeling the Upjohn Company and other companies did not clearly warn about the danger of Neomycin as an irrigant.

"Ms. Wells's surgeon used the Neomycin irrigation treatment during and after surgery, and when he sent her home from the hospital he had her continue the use of Neomycin irrigation.

"Neomycin is an antibiotic that belongs to the family of antibiotic drugs known as aminoglycosides. Medical science has established since the early forties and fifties that aminoglycoside antibiotics are ototoxic and many of them are ototoxic and nephrotoxic. Ototoxic means the drug has a toxic or harmful effect on the ability to hear. The drug causes damage to the eighth cranial nerve which connects the hearing apparatus in the ear to the brain. Once that drug gets into the system it is poorly eliminated through the kidneys. Nephrotoxic means the drug is toxic to or can cause damage to the kidneys.

"When a patient like Ms. Wells is given large doses of Neomycin in an irrigation solution, the danger is that large amounts of the Neomycin will be absorbed into the bloodstream and will go to the inner ear in the area known as the Organ of Corti. There the Neomycin resides for a long period of time. Once Neomycin gets into the inner ear in the area of the Organ of Corti, it is a protein inhibitor and attacks the hair-like nerve endings attached to the eighth cranial nerve. It destroys those hair-like nerve endings so the person cannot receive the sound wave impulses that send the hearing process from the inner ear to the brain.

"When the Neomycin is nephrotoxic it causes damage to the kidneys, making it hard for the body to eliminate the Neomycin. The Neomycin continues to build up in the person's system, making it more dangerous and more toxic. It is not unusual for hearing to be damaged many days or many weeks after treatment with Neomycin is discontinued. Most reported cases of Neomycin-induced deafness involve large doses of Neomycin. However there are cases reported in which Neomycin-deafness and tinnitus occurred when patients received the recommended or so-called therapeutic dosage of Neomycin. There is no known safe dosage of Neomycin. No known dosage of Neomycin invading the bloodstream and going to the inner ear can be guaranteed not to have ototoxic effects.

"At the time the case went to trial evidence clearly showed that no one, neither the surgeon nor the hospital, had informed her or warned her about the ototoxic and nephrotoxic side effects of Neomycin. Nor had her adult daughter who accompanied her to the hospital been warned about these dangers associated with Neomycin.

"When Ms. Wells was discharged, a member of the nursing staff followed the surgeon's orders to send several large containers of Neomycin solution home with Ms. Wells and instructed her daughter in applying the solution to her mother's shoulder until the Neomycin solution was used up. The nurse did not inform Ms. Wells or her daughter about the dangers and deafness side effects of Neomycin solution.

"Before Ms. Wells was admitted to the hospital she had normal hearing. During her hospital confinement, when she was receiving the Neomycin treatment, she did not demonstrate any signs or symptoms of any hearing loss. It was not until after she was released and her daughter completed the Neomycin irrigation that Ms. Wells started experiencing hearing loss.

"One of the phenomena associated with Neomycin-induced deafness is that the Neomycin stays in the inner ear for a prolonged period of time and even after the administration of the drug has been discontinued it continues to do its damage. That is what happened to Ms. Wells. The Neomycin was doing its damage to her inner ear while she was in the hospital. But it wasn't until after she went home and the home treatment with Neomycin was stopped that she began to realize she was losing her hearing.

"There are tests that could have and should have been done in the hospital to check her hearing at the higher

audiometric level. When Neomycin-deafness starts occurring it occurs in the upper or higher range of hearing first.
Not until it reaches the normal or lower ranges of hearing
can a person detect that they are losing their hearing.
Also, tests to detect the serum level of Neomycin in Ms.
Wells's bloodstream should have been done while she
was in the hospital. Had that been done, the doctors and
the pharmacy people could have realized she had an unac-
ceptably high level of Neomycin in her bloodstream which
would most likely cause her to experience a toxic effect if
the drug was continued. In addition, the hospital pharmacy did not monitor the use of the Neomycin drug in her
system along with other drugs being given to her, which
made the situation even worse.

"A week or so after the Neomycin irrigation was discontinued, Ms. Wells experienced a hearing problem and
tinnitus or ringing in her ears. This hearing problem progressed to total deafness. The tinnitus was a loud roaring
sound in her head which she described at the trial as being like sitting next to a giant jet engine.

"When Ms. Wells began experiencing hearing difficulty
she complained to her daughter, who arranged for her to
go and see her doctors. One of her doctors suspected that
she might be suffering from the ototoxic side effects of
antibiotics she was treated with. In the hospital she was
treated with Gentamicin as well as Neomycin. This form
of treatment is contraindicated because when a patient is
given two drugs of this type at the same time, in high
doses, the two act together to increase the toxicity.

"A very prominent medical doctor specializing in in-
fectious disease testified at the trial that Ms. Wells's
doctors were negligent in using Neomycin in high doses
and as an irrigant, that they should have realized that
Neomycin was unreasonably dangerous and should
never be used in treating infection of any type. This ex-
pert also testified that there were more effective drugs
that could have been safely used. A doctor of pharmacy,

a professor at the University of Texas School of Pharmacy, testified that Neomycin irrigation in large doses was the direct cause of Ms. Wells's deafness and tinnitus. He also testified that the hospital pharmacy was negligent in dispensing the Neomycin for use as an irrigant and failing to follow reasonable hospital pharmacy practice, failing to monitor the use and doses of Neomycin and failing to monitor Neomycin being used in conjunction with Gentamicin, another ototoxic aminoglycoside (category of antibiotic).

"The evidence in the case showed that the hospital pharmacy director did not file an adverse incident report with the FDA and none of the defendant doctors or the hospital notified the FDA of deafness and tinnitus in the Alberta Wells case.

"Literally thousands of doctors in America had been using Neomycin irrigationally to treat infections. Surgeons and hospitals continued to dispense Neomycin for irrigational use.

"At the time we went to trial in the case in 1985 Neomycin was still officially on the market.

"I was told that Ms. Wells was an outgoing and friendly person before this happened to her. Afterwards she became reclusive, irritable and frustrated at her inability to communicate and her inability to deal with tinnitus. The tinnitus was almost unbearable. It made her extremely depressed and at times suicidal.

"In the Alberta Wells case the jury rendered a verdict finding that negligence on the part of the hospital, the hospital pharmacy director, the treating physicians and the Upjohn drug company resulted in Ms. Wells's Neomycin-induced deafness and tinnitus from irrigational use of Neomycin for her shoulder wound. The verdict was in the amount of 1.5 million dollars.

"Over the years I represented three or four other folks who were injured by antibiotic therapy, including Neomycin treatment, that resulted in deafness. One was a woman in her mid thirties. She was injured in an automobile accident and suffered a broken hip. She was admitted to the hospital and developed an infection in the area where she had undergone surgery to repair her broken hip. Over a period of several months she received a combination of many antibiotics, including Neomycin. She suffered nerve deafness and tinnitus.

"In my opinion evidence has demonstrated that Neomycin Sulfate when used irrigationally has dangers that far outweigh its safety and effectiveness. There is no rational basis for keeping Neomycin on the market to be used irrigationally. It is a danger to Americans."

When your doctor prescribes cortisone, he or she may not advise you that cortisone can cause cataracts and other disorders, but many people are aware that cortisone can produce adverse reactions. Cortisone is commonly considered a dangerous drug, one to be administered only when there is no alternative. But there is no such common awareness that using loop diuretics and other medicines can make people deaf.

When new mothers used Parlodel to dry up their milk, the fatal strokes and heart attacks that resulted became celebrated cases. The FDA asked manufacturers to voluntarily remove Parlodel (bromocriptine mesylate) from use for anything except Parkinson's and other life-threatening diseases. When one drug company did not comply and new mothers continued to have seizures and strokes, a health advocacy group stepped in and sued the FDA to make it enforce its request about Parlodel.

But who defends the ear against ototoxicity? When prescriptions are filled, pharmacists paste warning labels on the consumers' containers. However, there is no warning label that says "may be ototoxic." The ear remains the neglected child of medicine.

This update details the dramatic damage Neomycin has done to ears. But deafness caused by Neomycin is only the tip of the iceberg. FDA files abound with cases of deafness caused by a tremendous battery of drugs. For every ototoxic drug listed in this chapter, there are victims.

Then there are my own files. Drawers filled with letters from people who suspect they are victims of ototoxic medicines: tetanus injections, Erythromycin, Neomycin sulfate, Gentamicin, aspirin—but people mainly wrote *antibiotic*. And most don't remember which antibiotic. There are only hazy recollections about the year. Many of these people have had hearing disorders since childhood, and parents, if they are living, do not remember the details. Some say the medication probably saved their lives, and of course no one can fault the use of medication in life-threatening situations. But all say they were never warned that the medicine might impair their hearing. Most are vague about the length of time it took for a medication to affect their hearing.

This is one of the problems with hearing impairment. It is difficult to pin down the exact time it happened, and equally difficult to associate the impairment with a specific medication that may have been taken at the time. If you are hit by a car, you and all the witnesses know a car hit you, causing your bruises and broken bones. If you are shot by a gun, you and all the witnesses know it was a gun that caused your wound. When you lose your hearing, neither you, nor witnesses in your family, nor friends, are likely to know exactly what hit you and when. Only in rare cases can people be precise about the ototoxicity of a specific pill or salve.

My neighbor Regina, who sits next to me at SHHH meetings, told me her doctor prescribed Neomycin sulfate tablets to be taken for a few days prior to surgery. Before taking the pills, she had a slight hearing loss, but functioned very well without hearing aids. The few days of medication gave her severe hearing loss. She said there had been no warning by her doctor and no warning on the prescription package. This was in the 1960s, and I wondered if that situation had been remedied. I knew that another friend's prescription package of Neomycin sulfate tablets had had no warning label pasted on it, but I thought perhaps the patient information leaflet that now accompanies many prescription drugs would contain a warning about ototoxicity.

I visited several neighborhood pharmacies to determine what patient information printout accompanied Neomycin sulfate tablets. At one pharmacy, the computer provided no patient information printout for Neomycin sulfate tablets but did provide a printout for Neomycin ointment. Though the printout warned of possible burning, redness, and stinging, there was not a word about potential harm to ears.

At another neighborhood pharmacy, the pharmacist gave me a lengthy patient information leaflet that had no warning about potential harm to one's hearing. The leaflet described side effects of Neomycin sulfate tablets, including nausea, diarrhea, dizziness, ringing in the ears, skin tingling, muscle twitching, or vaginal irritation or discharge. Not one word about hearing loss.

The pharmacist at another local pharmacy that is part of a large chain gave me a copy of the patient information leaflet* that accompanies Neomycin sulfate tablets and Neomycin ointment at his store; this leaflet did report that hearing trouble could be a side effect. After researching patient information leaflets in different parts of the country, I concluded that the information provided varies, and it is only by chance that the patient will get all the information needed to make a determination about a medicine's ototoxicity.

---

* Patient information leaflets supplied to pharmacies by First Databank in San Bruno, California, had proper warnings about hearing problems caused by Neomycin sulfate tablets and Neomycin ointment.

Both the hearing population and the already hearing-impaired population deserve complete and uniform access to the truth of what they are putting into and onto their bodies. Just as consumers must be informed when orange juice is made from concentrate, so consumers should be informed about the ototoxicity of prescription medications they are putting into and onto their bodies. There should be large red warning flags accompanying the pills, irrigators, and ointments that can make consumers candidates for the community that can hear no more.

The vulnerable ear needs defense before ototoxic medications reach the market. As Dr. Brummett related, newly developed drugs are not tested before being released to see if they will damage people's hearing. So in preparing this book for its paperback publication, I needed to know if there were still no requirements that prototype drugs be tested for ototoxicity.

My phone calls to the FDA asking about regulations requiring drug companies to test new, prototype drugs for ototoxicity produced a volume of reports intended to answer my query. In all these documents, I found no regulation requiring drug companies and independent laboratories to test new drugs for ototoxicity.

The FDA guidelines are concerned with establishing and maintaining good manufacturing practices so that drugs are produced under conditions that assure their integrity, in a qualified facility, with approved equipment, and using validated processes. When drug companies test new drugs on animals, it is easy to identify blindness, birth defects, and death factors. But unless the laboratory specifically addresses injury to the organ of hearing, how will it be able to determine if a new drug can cause deafness?

The words "toxic" and "safe" kept appearing in the many reports sent to me. The FDA is extremely concerned with the toxicity and safety of new drugs. But toxicity and safety are never related to the organ of hearing.

After studying the FDA reports, I wrote to Dr. Joseph DeGeorge, Supervisory Pharmacologist, Center for Drug Evaluation and Research. His gratifying response is the most promising sign that there may soon be FDA regulations that will help save the ears of our children:

> Thank you for your request regarding our requirements for the testing of new drugs for ototoxicity. We are currently involved in an effort to determine if current FDA guidelines for testing new drugs adequately address the potential of drugs to produce neurotoxicity.
>
> At the present, there are no specific requirements for testing neurotoxicity (including ototoxicity). . . . [However], we are aware of the relatively wide range of drugs which have produced ototoxicity, and would hope to include an assessment of ototoxicity in any new neurotoxicity guidelines which might be proposed. Your input in this area will add to the Agency's interest in this problem.

Those of us who inhabit the lonely world of hearing impairment are heartened that we stand on the threshold of an era that will identify deafening medications before they are put into human beings. And surely the fortunate Americans with normal hearing can rejoice that there may someday be FDA requirements that could save them from unnecessarily joining the world that can hear no more.

Chapter 14

Deafening Noise

When I was a child I sometimes heard the complaint, "That noise you're making is deafening!" I remember making the same complaint to my children when they and their friends ran through the house shouting. But the expression was merely a colloquialism. Who really thought noise was deafening? It was merely annoying. We know better now: there was much truth to those words.

Dr. Joseph Hawkins of the Kresge Hearing Research Institute at Ann Arbor, Michigan, relates presbycusis (sensorineural hearing impairment in the aged) to the noise factor. The findings of others indicate that the aged living in a quiet environment have fewer hearing disorders than those living in noisy cities. Dr. Hawkins discusses the connection between noise and hearing impairment:

"I came to the Kresge Hearing Research Institute at Michigan just as it was being started. One of my main interests has been the effects of noise on the hearing. The effect of intense noise on the ear was first revealed in Austria. There was the case of a deafened boilermaker who was killed by a train he had not heard approaching. A professor of otology named Habermann demonstrated changes in his inner ear as a result of his occupational noise exposure.

"In the 1940s at Harvard, I worked in Dr. Hallowell Davis's group with noise exposure effects on guinea pigs and also in human subjects. My colleagues and I exposed ourselves to a very high intensity of noise, which we thought was still in the nonharmful range. We eventually developed a considerable amount of hearing loss, probably attributable to that noise.

"I've worked with guinea pigs and monkeys that were exposed to noise and studied the effect on their hair cells, the organ of Corti, and the blood vessels of the inner ear. There is good evidence that the inner ear vessels constrict in response to noise.

"At New York University, New York City, and at the University of Michigan at Ann Arbor, I have worked with behavioral psychologists who train animals to do their own audiograms. We could then determine the amount of injury noise exposure caused to their hearing and to their inner ear structures. Dr. Lars Johnsson from Finland and I studied changes in human temporal bones of people exposed to intense noise in industry, hunting, war, and so forth."

With the truth known about deafening noise, how do people with hearing impairment prevent the noises of the '90s from further eroding their hearing? I use my hearing aids as plugs. When the band plays deafening music, when city streets threaten me, I use my aids—TURNED OFF. This is my best protection. Speechreading is also less complicated when there is no interference from deafening noise.

How does the hearing community protect itself? Today's teenagers are particularly at risk since they enjoy deafening music from headphones, stereos, and loud bands. Both loud music and environmental noise pollution are contributing to a generation who will be sadly

affected if they are not made aware of the truth about
deafening noise.

Keenan Wynn's Legacy for Young Ears

When I interviewed the late actor Keenan Wynn, he
addressed his concerns to young people who, like Wynn
himself as a youth, aren't careful enough:

"Noise. Loud noise was my problem. The damaging
noise of racing cars from the time I was fifteen until I was
in my early forties. My life was loud with that kind of
noise. Motorcycles and hydroplanes. That's what did it.
Because I didn't wear protection for my ears. And when
noise like that wrecks your hearing, there's nothing to be
done for it. Except, of course, hearing aids.

"I talk up about my hearing problem. I feel I must. For
the simple reason, if you have something wrong with you,
you don't go and hide it. That's dumb. I've always been
opposed to that. If you have a hearing problem, you have
to talk up. I've always been that way. I tell people immediately. And that makes it easier for me because then people
talk up and I can hear better.

"When I meet people who should wear hearing aids
and don't, I tell them I do. I try to tell them they should. I
say, 'I know why you're not wearing hearing aids. It's
because you're vain. Your vanity doesn't let you wear
them. You think it makes you look too old. Well, that's
ridiculous. It doesn't make you look too old. I've been
wearing these things for ten years, and they've had no
effect on my sex life whatsoever. Absolutely none! If you
hear better with hearing aids, you wear them. It's wrong
not to. You think the hearing aids make you look old? You
know what makes you look old? I'll tell you. When you
have to keep saying, "What? Wha? Who? Huh?" That's
what makes you look old. Not wearing a hearing aid.'

"I never worried that hearing impairment might interfere with my career as an actor. If it ever interfered, it would be my own fault. I tell the director right away that I wear hearing aids. If a particular part I am playing would make a hearing aid look out of place—for example, if the part is a Western set in 1840, before there were hearing aids—I can still manage. I will keep the aid in the one ear that is off camera. I will remove the aid from the ear that is on camera.

"Hearing impairment is not all downside. Many a good laugh has come from a harmless misunderstanding. One day I was talking with an actor friend of mine. He told me about having his twenty-two-year-old wife on the bedroom floor and then quickly laying a sensational forty-four-year-old gal in the closet.

"Of course, what he had actually said was that he didn't want to floor his twenty-two-year-old wife, who had come into the bedroom, so he quickly laid his forty-four special gat in the closet.

"I'm particularly interested in young people. I want them to know how I lost my hearing. I want them to be spared. So I do high school appearances. I've also made many educational tapes. I tell young people about the dangers of automobile noise and off-road vehicles, usually motorcycles. I warn them about factory noises and construction noises. I tell them they must wear protective head gear, ear protectors. And I tell these young people that very loud music can also be harmful. Hearing is a precious commodity. Once the damage is done, it's done!

"I love young people, but I'm interested in all people. I go to Rotary meetings and other luncheons and try to spread messages about hearing problems. I tell the audience that I'll be telling some funny jokes and if I see someone not laughing, I'll know it's because that person doesn't hear. Then I ask, 'How many people here wear hearing aids?' There will always be a few hands raised. Then I ask, 'How many people here need to be wearing

aids but don't?!' I get no raised hands on that question.
So I repeat that I'll know who they are when they don't
laugh at my jokes.

"Noise pollution is the one thing I'm most aware of. I
guess because it was a factor in my own hearing impairment. I try to get the message about hearing impairment
to as many young people as I can. When I talk at a high
school, I listen to the kids as they walk to the assembly
hall. No enthusiasm. They worry it's going to be a bore.
So right away I shock them out of their negative feelings. I
tell them about me and my problem and how it happened.
It's amazing. A good percent of them will stay after the
assembly just to talk with me. They want to save their
hearing. I make these appearances in schools all over the
country. I have to save that wonderful generation of
young people from making the mistakes I made."

Musicians and Hearing Loss

Musicians, physicians for musicians, and other music
professionals concerned about the damage to hearing
from exposure to excessive decibels founded H.E.A.R.
(Hearing Education and Awareness for Rockers). With an
office at the University of California-San Francisco Center
on Deafness, H.E.A.R. operates a national twenty-four-
hour hotline service that offers information, referrals, and
support network services and conducts a free hearing
screening program in the San Francisco Bay area.
H.E.A.R. has received international attention. It was the
focus of a government-sponsored Swedish film *Can't
Hear Your Knocking*. The Executive Director of H.E.A.R.,
Kathy Peck—a musician and song writer—has a 40 percent hearing loss aggravated by exposure to high volume.
She and Dr. Flash Gordon warn about the risks of exposure to excessively high volumes and offer information

about hearing protection. Among the musicians who speak out on hearing loss are Ray Charles, Peter Townshend of The Who, Soul Asylum's Dave Pirner, Ted Nugent, and Huey Lewis. In H.E.A.R. educational materials, Ted Nugent says, "My left ear is there primarily to balance my face, because it doesn't work at all. Now I always wear an earplug in my right ear." Huey Lewis adds, "Part of the power ritual at a live show is volume. But it should be monitored, out of concern for the audience."

The H.E.A.R. hotline number is 415-773-9590, or you can write to it at P.O. Box 460847, San Francisco, CA 94146. The H.E.A.R. offices are at the University of California-San Francisco Center on Deafness, 3333 California Street, Suite 10, San Francisco, CA 94118; voice telephone 415-441-9081, TTY 415-476-7600, fax 415-476-7113.

Chapter 15

Miracles: Little and Large

The Second Ear

People with hearing impairment wait endlessly for the big prize that will mean hearing happiness. Despite the daily challenges, the loneliness, the disappointments, those of us who have not given up—dropped out—face each day with fresh hope that a miracle will return us to the world of the hearing.

For many years such a miracle was the single-channel implant, which gave environmental sound to the profoundly impaired. Next came the implant with twenty-two channels, the implant that gave Charlotte Roth (see Chapter 7) a new lease on life. Then, on July 5, 1991, the *New York Times* featured another miracle; according to an article by Natalie Angier entitled "Experts Find Deaf Can Hear at High Ultrasonic Ranges," we may have a second ear:

> People can understand words spoken at high ultrasonic ranges once thought to be far beyond the capacity of human hearing, scientists have found. The ultrasonic speech must be conducted by an awkward laboratory device that transmits it through the bones of the skull, but when de-

livered in this manner even those who are profoundly deaf
can comprehend the words.

The findings raise the possibility that people may have
a second, previously unknown acoustical organ that is distinct from the cochlea of the inner ear, which detects the
sounds of everyday life. And they suggest a new approach
for designing devices to help those who can hear little or
nothing in normal audio ranges.

The results of the research were reported today in the
journal *Science*.

Deaf Respond to Sound   "Clearly there is a system that
will respond to sound even in deaf people whose cochleas
have been badly destroyed," Dr. Martin L. Lenhardt of the
Medical College of Virginia in Richmond, the lead author
of the report, said Wednesday in an interview. "That
suggests there is some compensatory mechanism at
work."

But scientists do not know what kinds of deafness
might be helped by the new approach.

Much remains to be done before any sort of hearing aid
based on the new approach will be available, but the researchers hope eventually to have a little patch the size of
a quarter that can be taped to the neck to translate normal
speech into ultrasonic tones for those who are partly or
wholly deaf. The research was financed in part by Hearing
Innovations, a company in Tucson, Ariz., that holds pa-
tents on the method.

Other doctors who have heard about the new results
say they are cautiously impressed, but they add that they
need far more data to be thoroughly convinced.

"Difficult to Understand"   "It's an intriguing idea, but
one would have to say this goes very much against the
conventional wisdom," said Dr. Noel L. Cohen, chairman
of the department of otolaryngology at New York University Medical Center in Manhattan and one of the nation's

leading authorities in the study of hearing impairments. "From what appears in the paper, it's difficult to understand exactly what they're claiming their results are. It could be very exciting, a really major breakthrough, but on the other hand it could be pie in the sky."

Researchers have been dabbling since the 1940s with comparative studies of how different animals respond to ultrasonic frequencies. Dogs can hear extremely high-pitched tones, as can many small mammals, reptiles, and insects, but humans were thought to be limited to sounds below 20,000 cycles a second. Standard human speech falls between 300 and 3,000 cycles a second.

Some experiments indicated that humans could detect tones slightly above the uppermost range if the sound were conveyed so close to the head that the bones were vibrated. But scientists thought such ultrasonic noises would be perceived as nothing more than monotonous squeals and thus could hardly serve to convey information like speech.

But while pursuing an effort to help the endangered sea turtle by deterring it from treacherous beaches through the use of ultrasonic alarms, Dr. Lenhardt said he found he could discern considerable modulations and tonal differences in frequencies supposedly way above his hearing capacity, in the range of 30,000 cycles a second and beyond.

He said he and his colleagues could hear the ultrasounds by using a device the size of a videocassette recorder that is attached to the head and vibrates it extremely rapidly. When the head is vibrated at such high frequencies, Dr. Lenhardt said, "you perceive the vibrations as sound."

Going further, the researchers tried translating words into these same high frequencies and conducting them through the vibrating device. They found they could easily make out the ultrasonic tones as distinct words.

"It Sounded Like Speech" "What amazed me is that
when I first heard it, it sounded like speech," Dr. Lenhardt said. "It was a high-pitched squeaky kind of sound,
like an old-time voice synthesizer, but we hadn't thought
we'd be able to recognize any speech at all."

The researchers then tested a group of people whose
hearing capacity ranged from excellent to non-existent.
The people were given a list of six words and were told
they would be hearing one of them. The words were
closely related phonetically, like socks, rocks, and fox.

The subjects were told to point to a picture indicating
the word they had just heard. Young adults with excellent
normal hearing also did well in the ultrasonic, picking the
right picture more than 80 percent of the time. Older
adults, who had lost much of the upper ranges of their
normal hearing—as commonly happens with age—did not
seem to suffer a similar decrement in their ultrasonic
hearing, scoring almost as well as their youthful counter-
parts.

Most encouraging to the researchers was the performance of three people who were profoundly deaf. They
picked the proper word 40 to 60 percent of the time.

Dr. Lenhardt suggests that another organ in the inner
ear, the saccule, may be involved in responding to ultrasound. Although better known for its role in controlling
balance and the perception of movement, the saccule, a
tiny gel-filled structure, could also act like a high-frequency tuning fork, picking up ultrasound vibrations and
transmitting them along the same pathway as signals
travel from the cochlea to the brain. Thus, the vibrations
from the saccule could, under certain circumstances, end
up being perceived by the brain as sound.*

Programming Aids to Individual Needs

People with hearing disabilities wait on tenterhooks for the miracle that nature and auditory scientists may spring on us at any time. Until this happens there are smaller miracles for ears that need more than conventional hearing aids.

Several years ago multiprogrammable hearing instruments were introduced. Just as eyeglasses are made to accommodate the individual eye, so too are hearing aids programmed for the individual ear. Basic programming is done by an audiologist who studies the patient's audiogram and then tests various settings under various conditions with the patient. The professional program for some programmable aids is set into a small ($2\frac{1}{2}''$ by $4''$ by $\frac{1}{2}''$) remote control unit that sends signals to the patient's hearing aids. The unit can be carried in a pocket or purse.

Once the audiologist's setting in the remote control unit is locked in place the user can make adjustments by pressing any one of four buttons to accommodate various environments. Adjustments can be made for a noisy social event, a restaurant, an industrial environment, and so on. Then another button can be pressed when the environment changes to a quiet, well-insulated area. Adjustments can be made for better hearing in a musical environment, a multiconversational environment, and a one-on-one conversation, all either out-of-doors or indoors. Programmable aids accommodate the wide range of environmental changes the ear is subjected to each day. The remote control unit is just what it is called—remote control; that is, once an environment is chosen and a button is pressed to send an appropriate signal to the hearing aids, the aids will obey that signal until a different button is pressed. A person can go for a walk on a quiet country road with a companion and leave the remote control unit at home if it has been programmed to accommodate the

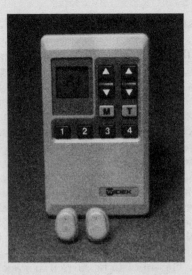

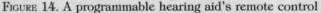

FIGURE 14. A programmable hearing aid's remote control

environment of a quiet country road. During the walk without the remote control unit on hand, no environmental program changes can be made. However, the hearing aids, like conventional aids, can be adjusted to make sounds louder or softer.

Programmable aids improve telephone comprehension when they are used with the unit's telephone button and are extremely helpful when used in combination with other telephone assistive devices like the Comtek Adapter. Programmable aids are of immense value not only for mildly and moderately impaired ears but for severely damaged ears as well. They are available in behind-the-ear and in-the-ear hearing aids.

The cost of the remote control unit plus two hearing aids is approximately twice the cost of two conventional hearing aids, but the benefits are amazing. With programmable hearing aids I can once again discern many area speech patterns, a miraculous feat for my severely impaired ears. The improvement in my "out of sight" speech comprehension (discrimination) astounds audiologists and ear doctors. (See this book's Directory of Resources for a list of facilities that provide total service, which includes programmable hearing aids, or that can recommend facilities with total service in your area. The directory also includes a list of companies that manufacture programmable aids.)

FM Hearing Aids

I recently interviewed audiologist Steven Malawer at the Hearing and Speech Center at Long Island Jewish Medical Center. Steven fitted me with the one Free Ear, an FM hearing aid, available at the Hearing Aid Dispensary. The Free Ear microphone was clipped to his shirt and I could hear him with amazing clarity. Not a word was lost to my severely impaired ear when I looked away from Steven's mouth to make notes about what he was saying. And this was quite miraculous since I must rely on my eyes to speechread even when I use two traditional high-power aids in the same environment.

In his room in the hearing aid dispensary, Steven sat a long table length away from me discussing the newest assistive listening devices, which were spread out on the table between us. He also described listening devices that would be available in the near future. He started off by saying, "I think one of the first people to make the public aware of Behind the Ear (BTE) FM hearing aids was Miss America. At a meeting of the American Academy of Audiologists she explained why she wore the FM hearing aids when she was crowned Miss America. When she dances she needs to hear the introduction to the music in order to begin and get the timing of her dance right. Once she starts, it doesn't matter whether or not she hears since she has the dance memorized. When she danced at various pageants, she would come on stage and immediately people would clap, making it impossible for her to hear the start of the music when she wore traditional hearing aids. This threw her timing off. Then she learned about FM hearing aids.

"With BTE FM she switched to the FM only, which meant she did not pick up any outside sounds. She would only hear what the microphone was delivering. The microphone was hooked right into the music machine so she would not hear anything else around her except for the music. The audio system, a musician or a machine, would have to be wearing the sending equipment.

"Two FM behind-the-ear models are now available. One, made by AVR Communications Ltd., is called the Extend-Ear. The other is the Free Ear. Free Ear is produced by Phonic Ear, which no longer produces standard hearing aids. Free Ear is distributed through Oticon. Both of these systems have the feature of an FM receiving unit located in the hearing aid itself. In the Free Ear there is a small antenna attached to the aid. You can feel it if you reach back behind your ear. It's like a little string. Formerly you had to have an FM receiver that you would wear on your belt or on a body pack. That would have been unacceptable for Miss America.

"FM hearing aids are mainly used in a classroom. The teacher wears the microphone and the student wears the FM receiver. FM aids are a very hot topic. They are not only recommended for hearing-impaired adults and children but for 'attention deficit children.' The FM system shuts out all distracting sounds. The person talking can be in the next room and the FM hearing aid wearer will understand what is being said.

"The major difference between these two available FM hearing aids is that with the Free Ear, the person speaking must wear the microphone. If there are many people in a room and the hearing-impaired person wearing a Free Ear wants to communicate with them all, the microphone must be passed from speaker to speaker, must be attached, released, and attached. This means that speakers talking to people using the Free Ear will have to participate physically in the process.

"With the Extend-Ear, all the work can be done by the hearing aid wearer who holds the microphone—a single stick about the size of a half a dozen pencils wrapped together with a rubber band. It is very portable. The person with hearing impairment can manage the entire situation, holding the microphone near one speaker and then moving it to another speaker. Of course, some speakers may offer to hold the microphone while they are communicating with the person who is hearing impaired, but that is at his or her option.

"I think that as more people use FM hearing aids, public lectures will accommodate them. At the beginning of a public lecture everyone will turn onto the same channel. The lecturer will tell people to put hearing aids on a certain channel and everyone will adjust their FM receiver to be on the same frequency. I believe the FM hearing aid is the wave of the future."

The cost of two FM hearing aids plus clip-on or portable microphone/transmitter can range from $2,500 to $4,000.

Miraculous Aid for an Uncommon Disorder

Consulting ear doctors does not always present a solution for a hearing disorder. In the case of a little girl who became unresponsive after she recovered from the measles at age three, conventional hearing aids were not helpful. Dr. Charles I. Berlin, Director of Louisiana State University Medical Center's Ear, Nose and Throat Department's Kresge Hearing Research Laboratory of the South, made the first precise diagnosis and helped develop a proper aid for the unusual disorder, called residual high-frequency hearing. An article appearing in *Time* magazine (September 13, 1982) entitled "Help for High-Frequency Hearers" describes the "translator" device Dr. Berlin helped develop to bring hearing to those with this disorder:

> After a bout with measles, three-year-old Karyl Ann Mirmelstein of Newport News, Va., seemed strangely unresponsive. Her mother consulted a number of doctors, who variously attributed the child's behavior to sibling rivalry with her baby sister, a learning disability, and even mental retardation. "I knew this couldn't be true," says Rona Mirmelstein. "I could see that Kam was very bright, perhaps more so than most children." Yet it was not until Kam was six that doctors acknowledged that her problem was her hearing. The results of an elaborate series of auditory tests were perplexing. While Kam could hear the sharp sound of a telephone ringing or a door slamming, she did not respond to subtler noises. A standard hearing aid was recommended, but Kam refused to wear it, relying instead on lipreading. Eventually, she graduated from college, married a lawyer from Long Island, N.Y, and resigned herself to being an "audiological enigma."
>
> Then, at age 27, she met Charles I. Berlin, an audiologist who heads the Kresge Hearing Research Laboratory of the South in New Orleans. Using special equipment, Berlin was able for the first time to provide a precise diagnosis of Kam's problem: "ultra-audiometric" hearing, that is, the capacity to hear, but only at extremely high frequencies.
>
> People with ultra-audiometric hearing, says Berlin, are usually born with full-range hearing, but become deaf in the lower registers after suffering a high fever, virus or meningitis in childhood. Some have an extended upper au-

ditory range and can hear dog whistles or the shrill hiss of a department-store electronic security system. Their problem, as in Kam's case, generally goes undetected because of inadequate testing. Most testing devices do not produce sounds above a certain frequency, Berlin says, "and it is precisely at this cutoff that ultra-audiometric patients begin hearing." Worse still, ultra-audiometrics may lose what hearing they have if they use conventional hearing aids, says Berlin. "The aids can cause overstimulation or acoustic trauma."

Kam's case was one of several that prompted Berlin to begin developing a hearing device that would "translate" low-frequency sounds into the range at which ultra-audiometrics could hear them. With help from engineers at the Illinois firm of Knowles Electronics, he produced a miniature magnetic earphone with two channels. One channel amplifies high-pitched sounds: the other shifts lower pitches upward into the range heard by ultra-audiometrics. The earphone is wired to a battery pack and microphone.

For Kam, the device opened up a bustling world, both raucous and musical. Recounting her first exposure in her diary, she wrote: "All voices sounded like jabberwocky because they were so different." As she adjusted, however, she found that "I was able to understand my cousin despite the fact that he has a low voice and a mustache." Later, she rediscovered music: "I put *Exodus* on the stereo. So stirring was the music that I suddenly began to cry in an almost hysterical way. The beauty of the sound was almost torture—I simply couldn't get enough of it."

There are about 20 million hearing-impaired Americans, and Berlin guesses that as many as 20,000 could be helped by his device. To find them, he has begun testing students in schools for the hearing-impaired. In addition, eight free ultra-audiometric testing centers have been established across the country, along with a collect-call hot line (301-897-8682) to field questions about the condition. So far, Berlin and his colleagues have uncovered 167 potential patients, 37 of whom have received translators paid for by contributions to a fund started by Kam's mother. None is more delighted than Kam, who, at 32, has become a teacher of hearing-impaired adolescents: "My hearing aid has given me a chance to have a profession. I never could have done it without one."*

Finger Magic

A recent article in *Business Week* entitled "Now, the Deaf Can Listen with Their Fingers" describes a newly invented device that enables the deaf to hear with their fingers:

> Today, many blind people use their fingers to read. Tomorrow, deaf people may do the same to hear. That's because Australian scientists, led by Robert Cowen at the University of Melbourne, have developed a Walkman-size gadget dubbed the Tickle Talker.
>
> Its microphone listens to speech, and a digital-signal processing chip sorts out sounds, particularly those that are hard to distinguish by lipreading. Each sound triggers an electrical signal that is sent to a specific spot on ring-like bands worn on the fingers of one hand. For example, "s" and "z" sounds are felt as a tickling sensation on the outside of the little finger.
>
> After a couple of weeks of training, one severely deaf lipreading adult scored 100% in word- and sentence-comprehension tests, up from 60% and 75%, respectively, with just a hearing aid. Another adult, who is profoundly deaf—a hearing aid is of no benefit—nearly doubled his

scores from levels of 30% to 50% for words, sentences, and consonant sounds.*

Regeneration of Neurosensory Mechanisms

Newly resourceful, Cynthia has found employment in a school with a class for hearing-handicapped children. She takes them on long walks through a park area and points out birds. She talks and signs in manual alphabet about bird song they will never hear unless—and this is the critical word—unless remarkably promising progress is made in research on deafness. Cynthia does not want to give her students false hope, so she tells them cautiously about experimentation that is in its infancy. She wants them to be aware of the good things the future holds for the 17 million people with sensorineural impairment.

Cynthia's message to the children comes from the following article, entitled "Regeneration of Neurosensory Mechanisms," found in *A Report of the Task Force on the National Strategic Research Plan* (1989), published by the National Institute on Deafness and Other Communication Disorders:

> Sensorineural or "nerve" deafness has been considered irreversible because the production of the permanent sensory and nerve cells of the ear normally ceases before birth (in the fetus). Recent basic research with animals, however, has shown that under certain conditions sensory cell production can be reactivated in mature damaged ears. It is also known that these regenerated cells contribute to a recovery of hearing. Study of the cellular mechanisms and the molecular control of this self-repair process is readily amenable to methods of modern biotechnology.

* Reprinted from *Business Week,* December 16, 1991, by special permission. Copyright © 1991 by McGraw-Hill, Inc.

Basic elucidation of the process should lead to therapeutic advances.

It is reasonable to expect that within the foreseeable future the progenitors of regenerated sensory cells will be cloned from animals and that the product will become available for the development of pharmacological agents for controlling regenerative cell replacement and auditory recovery. In addition, the natural molecular triggers for sensory cell growth and inhibition and the potential occurrence of spontaneous sensory cell regeneration in species more closely related to humans should be extensively evaluated.

The realization of clinical gains from this research is likely to require 10 to 20 years of sustained investigation, but the potential benefits are great. For 80 percent of the 28 million Americans affected by hearing impairment, their loss is currently irreversible, due to inner ear deafness. The studies proposed here suggest that this type of deafness might not have to be considered permanent.

The information Cynthia shares with her hearing-disabled students also comes from my conversations with doctors in research laboratories. Dr. Berlin told me, "Research in this field of regeneration of neurosensory mechanisms shows that regeneration occurs almost exclusively in birds rather than in mammals. Dr. Webster, in our laboratory, has shown that certain strains of deaf mice have some regeneration at the low-frequency zone of hair cells. But we're not sure that these regenerated hair cells are useful to the mice. However, a lot of laboratories around the country are studying regeneration to see how it can be applied in the mammalian ear." Dr. Hawkins also discussed the issue of regeneration with me: "I would say that regeneration is not inconceivable. I am aware of regeneration of neurosensory mechanisms in birds and chicks, so regeneration of neurosensory mechanisms in the mammalian ear may not be entirely out of the question."

A Most Achievable Miracle: The Loop

A hospital can be a hearing-impaired person's nightmare. Compounding the pain, the fear, and the anxiety of illness is the dread of not understanding what a nurse or doctor must explain. Not understanding these vital words can lead to thinking the worst. Hospital programs designed for people with hearing impairment are rare. And even these programs, while they are to be applauded, are not a total solution.

People with hearing impairment dream of "the day of the loop" (see Chapter 5 for a description of this sound-amplifying device). At a cost of $700, perhaps less, architects' plans for new hospital construction could include one room with loop equipment (until that ideal construction, hospitals could own one portable loop). For a small investment of $700 by the hearing world's health and emergency facilities, people with hearing impairment could activate the T switch on their hearing aids and be tuned into life-supporting words.

The loop can bring life-supporting words to arenas other than health facilities. My article, "Let Them Have a Fair Hearing," in the *Cleveland Plain Dealer* (September 19, 1990) describes the plight of two women in a court of law without benefit of a loop:

> Hearing-impaired people are greatly disadvantaged in courts. In these large public structures, where there are no soft, high-pile carpets and furniture fabrics to absorb background noise, hearing-impaired who serve as witnesses or are themselves plaintiffs or defendants have difficulty understanding judges, lawyers, and other litigants.

Americans take pride in our small-claims courts that give easy and inexpensive access to an official judical decision and/or settlement. These courts are designed to give every person his or her day in court. For the hearing-impaired, however, there is one large fault in the design.

My friend Helen sued in small claims court when she had continuous leakage and water damage after a new roof was put on her small house. The roofing company had been unresponsive to her numerous phone calls and letters. Helen is articulate and well-educated; she was most competent to argue her own case. Everything was in Helen's favor—everything but her ears that are severely impaired.

It was impossible for Helen to understand the fast-paced, deep-voiced conversation between the arbitrator and the man from the roofing company. Compounding this difficulty, the roofer had a heavy beard, making it impossible for Helen to read his lips. She finally settled for a fraction of the amount to which she felt entitled.

My neighbor Rita had her unhappy day in a civil court. Rita, also hearing impaired, had been subpoenaed to serve as a witness and wanted to do her public duty efficiently and honestly. Unable to understand what the judge and the lawyers were saying, Rita explained her hearing impairment and asked the judge to have the lawyers stand directly in front of her so she could read their lips. The judge refused, explaining that the attorneys must stand farther back to give the jury an unobstructed view of them.

Rita then asked for an oral interpreter. The judge said he could not make such provision without postponing the case. Rita was quite upset. Her lawyer told her that what mattered was what she said, not what she heard.

Rita could not accept this. She told the judge and her lawyer, "There are interpreters for people who speak a foreign language; why not one for someone with hearing impairment?"

Her comment was ignored.

Rita became increasingly nervous. The judge, unwilling to postpone the case, allowed the lawyers to stand where Rita could see much, though not all, of what was being said. Her day in court left Rita nerve-racked and troubled because she felt she had not been a totally competent witness.

There is equipment called a "loop" that would have made it possible for both Rita and Helen to hear properly. "Loop" wire, clipped to the perimeter of a room, works in conjunction with hearing aids set on their "T" telephone position. This system eliminates background noise interference and brings voices to the impaired ear with such clarity that the impaired ear has almost normal comprehension or discrimination.

The loop would solve a serious problem for the large community of hearing-impaired people. One out of 10 Americans has some degree of hearing impairment; 7.2 million have significant bilateral hearing loss and have difficulty understanding what is said in normal conversation. This large segment of the population depends on assistive aids like the loop.

The loop would also be a budget benefit for the courts. The loop, for a one-time expenditure of $700, would eliminate the continuing expense and inconvenience of postponing cases until oral interpreters are hired. One portable loop could service an entire complex of courts.

It is the hope that the Americans With Disabilities Act of 1990 will be implemented to require that future court buildings install permanent loops and existing courts use portable loops, so hearing-impaired people have equal opportunity to a fair day in court.

In some Scandinavian countries it is required that state churches be "looped." Most public buildings in these countries are looped. Then why not here? Why not for me and all my friends with hearing impairment? We dream of theaters with one row looped, of looped schools, lecture halls—all public buildings.

Because people with hearing impairment experience difficulty understanding spoken communication in buses, trains, trolleys, cruise ships, the Mobiloop Hearing Assistance System was developed. Mats have also been developed to help people with hearing impairment understand the spoken word. The 3-D Loop Mat can be placed under any nonmetallic flooring surface. For information about these miraculous loop systems, call 800-438-5667 or 800 GET-LOOP.

Chapter 16

To Do and Not to Do: How to Manage Hearing Impairment

Hints, Caveats, Examples, and Anecdotes in Chapters 1–14: Guides for People with Hearing Impairment and for the Hearing

This chapter summarizes the ways, both little and large, people with hearing impairment can help themselves. And it is a ready reminder for the hearing who want to participate and assist with the daily challenges their hearing-disabled friends and family members face.

Guide for People with Hearing Impairment

Patience is essential for people with hearing impairment. The best assistive aids for ears, unlike assistive aids for eyes, do not place the impaired ear on a par with the normal ear. At best, people with hearing impairment can narrow the gulf that keeps them a world apart from the hearing.

I remind myself about this need for patience when I attend an evening of bridge with a small group of friends and bridge teacher friend Jules Dendy. For the hour lecture by Jules, I remove my hearing aids and wear special hearing molds attached to my Williams Sound PFM Receiver; Jules keeps the Williams Sound PFM transmitter and microphone in his shirt pocket.

Reception is excellent. The only one in the room I am tuned into is Jules, so there is no background noise interference. Using my eyes and the Williams sound system, I understand almost every word Jules says about the bridge convention he is teaching (a few words do escape me when Jules turns his head away from where I sit or when he rattles his notes).

If Jules were talking about a current news topic or relating an uncomplicated anecdote, I would understand satisfactorily enough, but the bridge lecture is mathematical. Jules is dealing with numbers and the patterns of distribution of these numbers. I concentrate so intently on each word he speaks that it is not easy for me to process them. The meaning of what he says drifts away. Intent upon hearing each word, the intricacies and complexities of a new bridge convention are lost. It is as though my mind has wandered. Of course, good friend Jules has patience and would repeat the points he has made, but I am not going to make this a late evening for my group of friends. I remind myself that nothing is perfect, that I do not want to be a dropout, that I will read Jules's notes another time, that I will try to have a mile of patience with my unfortunate ears.

Acknowledge your own impairment; don't wait for others to do it for you (Chapter 1).

Make clear rules when you have passengers in your car (Chapter 3).

Educate your telephone companions about your special need for keeping conversations simple, about your need for special telephone language, and about your problems with certain telephones (Chapter 2).

Express gratitude to thoughtful hearing people (Chapter 3).

Binaural assistance helps more than twice as much. (Chapter 10).

Explain body language and need for light on lips of the speaker to the hearing who want to communicate (Chapters 1–3).

Avoid further damage to your ears (Chapters 1, 11, and 12).

Give up old habits that create problems for you, for example, calling to others in other parts of the house (Chapter 2).

Cultivate activities that don't require acute hearing— sports, cards, arts and crafts, gardening, exercise groups, dance groups (Chapter 6).

Remain aware of limitations to avoid embarrassment. For example, don't enter the room talking; others may be in conversation or using a telephone.

Look at faces in a group before speaking to avoid breaking into a conversation.

Avoid danger by being constantly aware of limitations. When faucets are opened, remain at the site until the tap is shut off. It's easy to forget, and impaired ears may not hear running water. Impaired ears need more caution than normal ears. Impaired ears may not hear boiling pots or sizzling foods, so it may be unsafe to cook and do other chores at the same time.

When memory fails, people with hearing impairment won't get the same assistance a hearing person gets. If you forget someone's name during group conversation, there may be no point waiting for the name to be repeated; try writing a note to a friend sitting close by.

Pronunciation of the names of new personalities or products may be impossible to learn from radio or TV. Watch for newspaper notes about pronunciation of new names. Good friends can help. Don't hesitate to ask.

Don't shy away from socializing; you may lose the art of conversation.

Help hearing friends and family learn how to interact with you. Don't lose heart when it is necessary to remind the hearing.

Communicative interaction is almost always a challenge. Be persistent about making person-to-person relationships work.

Assistive aids must be studied, practiced with, and prodded along in order to have them do their jobs properly. One of my most effective telephone aids, the Comtek unit, gave me no help initially. The device is so powerful it tuned me into radio airwaves that obscured the voice at the other end of my wire. A phone call to Mr. Belgique at Comtek solved the problem; "Remove the M crystal," he told me. At once I was able to have a telephone conversation without the interference that supersensitive crystal brought in. People with hearing impairment must never give up; they must never give in to the constant challenge.

Don't accept the negative. My friend Cynthia asked her ear doctor what he thought about programmable aids. "Not for you," he said. "You have flat loss. They'll do you no good." Cynthia went to a meeting where an audiologist spoke about programmable (digital) aids. Cynthia showed him her audiogram, and he told her, "Don't waste your time and money." No longer the dropout, Cynthia decided to try them anyway. To everyone's amazement, these very special aids improved her comprehension by 35 percent.

Guides for the Hearing

The hearing can help once they understand the singular problems of impairment.

One evening I telephoned a woman friend to confirm an appointment with her and two other women. My husband would be taking the four of us to a neighborhood restaurant on the coming Sunday. I was hooked into complicated equipment that is a blessing but, like all assistive aids, not perfect. When I told my friend that my husband would be taking the four of us to dinner the coming Sunday, she thanked me, and I thought she said, "So he'll be dating four women." I answered, "Yes, he probably won't get a word in edgewise."

Apparently, my friend had not said my husband would be dating four women. She repeated with a few quick words, and all I understood was "four." From the far end of the room my husband heard my friend's voice on the phone, and he held up four fingers. "I know, four," I told him. Impatiently, he approached the telephone and wrote AUGUST FOURTH.

My friend had taken our conversation an unnecessary step forward. When I said this coming Sunday, she added, "Sunday the fourth." My husband could not see into my processing mind to understand that I had missed many words and had related the number four to the number of women we would be.

It's important for the hearing to keep reminding themselves that just as their minds may sometimes not focus, so too a hearing-impaired person's mind may fail to focus or process correctly.

Hearing people should not make determinations for people with hearing impairment (Chapters 1 and 5).

You are not being tuned out by the hearing-impaired—you are not heard (Chapter 4).

People with hearing impairment cannot help using too much or too little voice (Chapter 4).

Your words can be seen, so don't be tempted to talk about a person with hearing impairment in that person's presence. Most hearing-impaired people speechread.

Use special consideration when walking on a busy thoroughfare with a hearing-impaired person (Chapter 3).

Address the person with hearing impairment directly, even when he or she is accompanied by a hearing person (Chapter 7).

Servicepeople, salespeople—everyone—should keep in mind that those who do not understand or seem not to be listening may have a hearing disability (Chapter 3).

Dentists and doctors, help your patient see your words (See Chapter 3). If you wear a protective mask, see-through models are available.*

Give up the old habit of calling out from another part of the house if you live with a hearing-impaired person (Chapter 2).

You may not realize how upsetting it is for people with hearing impairment to be told, when they do not understand what is being said, "It's not important" or "I'll tell you when I see you." These telephone comments by the hearing can be avoided by keeping phone conversations brief and simple.

Substitute a different word when a hearing-impaired person fails to understand; repeating a word is not as helpful. My grandson Adam substituted instinctively when he was four years old. Substituting words for the misunderstood words is an excellent way to communicate with people who are hearing impaired.

Take care when expressing affection. Hearing aids whistle when they are touched. Hearing aids can be painful when the impaired ear gets a loving embrace.

Please protect the impaired ear. Hearing-impaired ears need protection from respiratory infection. The person with hearing impairment may not recognize from the sound of a voice that a person has a cold. It is a kindness to announce a respiratory infection.

Leaning close to the impaired ear is rarely helpful. Peo-

---

* Fluid-shield procedure masks, manufactured by Baxter, are available at dental supply houses. A box of 25, for $28.99, will make you a good friend to your patients with hearing impairment.

ple with hearing impairment must see the mouth that is speaking.

Use body language. My granddaughter Anna uses her body like a ballerina to help me over hurdles with language. All hearing people can't be ballerinas, but most everyone can learn body movement to help clarify words misunderstood by people with hearing impairment.

Announce your willingness to help, and people with hearing impairment will clue you in. Hearing friends and family members can learn from each other. My youngest grandchild, Andrew, has learned from his sister, brother, and cousins how to make himself understood. He uses his mouth and body to make sure his grandmother is a full part of his world.

Face the person with impairment whenever voice is used, a most difficult behavior change to remember. At times this facing requires extreme discipline: For example, when a group includes a person with hearing impairment, it is helpful when the speaker faces the person with impairment even when the question or answer is directed from one hearing person to another hearing person.

When chatting on the telephone with a loved one of the person with hearing impairment, keep the receiver away from your mouth so the impaired person can at least be partially clued into the sense of a phone call he or she would give a piece of life to be a direct party to (Chapter 2).

On the Plus Side

Talking with Cynthia and others in my SHHH group, I developed a list focusing on the way daily life can be easier for people with hearing impairment and on some of the pluses of hearing impairment. For example: People with hearing impairment aren't frightened by squeaking floorboards at night. People with hearing aids have ear protection from flying insects and particles. People with hearing aids can easily tune out unwanted noise.

People with hearing impairment can make their own special plus lists. People with hearing impairment can make their own happy endings.

Directory of Resources

Assistive Aids

People with hearing impairment must experiment to learn about assistive aids that will accommodate their individual disorder. Some Self Help for Hard of Hearing People, Inc. (SHHH) groups or chapters have assistive aid displays. Organizations like the League for the Hard of Hearing also have large displays. The Williams Sound Corporation, AT&T's National Special Needs Center, and Radio Shack will send catalogs describing assistive aids. People with hearing impairment can find many assistive devices for their special needs at one of the more than 7,000 Radio Shack stores. Assistive aid centers, where equipment may be tried, can be located by contacting SHHH's national headquarters, local hospitals with hearing and speech centers, or the associations and organizations listed in this directory.

For information about most assistive aids, call AT&T Special Needs Center (toll free): 800-233-1222. Ma Bell is a true mother, offering a free thirty-day trial with a wide assortment of aids—everything from telecaption decoders to light alerts to the common handsets, bell and voice amplifiers, and the like.

A most effective aid for my severely impaired ears is the Williams Personal FM System. With receiver in one pocket and microphone clipped to my lapel, I can join a conversation in a noisy environment. I am no longer "out of it." Yes, I miss some words, but I understand enough to keep me part of the hearing world. With conventional hearing aids, restaurants are generally off limits to my ears. With programmable aids or the Williams Personal FM System, I am no longer a restaurant dropout.

The following list offers only a partial picture of what is out there waiting to assist impaired ears. No list can be complete. Even at this moment, new pieces of assistive equipment are being developed.

Hearing Aids

T (telephone) switches are available with most behind the ear hearing aids. High-tech programmable hearing aids, which are sophisticated state-of-the-art aids, are tailored to fit the individual problem and have an approximate cost range of $2,000 to $3,500. The names and phone numbers of some of the companies that manufacture programmable aids are:

Resound (800-248-HEAR)
Siemens (908-562-6600)
Starkey (800-441-1395)
3M (800-882-3M3M)
Widex (718-482-1844)

FM Hearing Aids

FREE EAR: Phonic Ear (707-769-1110)
EXTEND-EAR: AVR Sonovation (800-462-8336)

Hearing-Dog Center

Dogs are trained to respond to smoke alarms, crying babies, alarm clocks, telephones, doorbells, buzzers, and knockers.

Delta Society/American Humane Hearing Dog Resource Center; phone: 800-869-6898 voice/TTY.

Listening Systems: Individual

LISTENAIDER: Nasta Industries, C.F.A.-2030 Green Street, Philadelphia, PA 19130; phone: 215-698-2121; cost: approximately $30

WILLIAMS SOUND PERSONAL FM SYSTEM: Williams Sound Corporation; 10399 W. 70th St., Eden Prairie, MN 55344-3459; phone: 800-328-6190; cost: approximately $530; also available nationally through audiologists

PHONIC EAR FM SYSTEM: Phonic Ear, 250 Camino Alto, Mill Valley, CA 94941; fax: 415-332-3085; phone: 415-385-4000; cost: approximately $1100

POCKETALKER: AT&T Special Needs Center; 800-233-1222; cost: approximately $140

TELEX: Telex Communications, Inc., 9600 Aldrich St., Minneapolis, MN 55344; phone: 800-328-6190; cost: approximately $400

SONY STEREO HEADPHONES: The high-power headphones MDR 7506 that can be used to hear movies on airplanes were first called to my attention by Ruth Shapiro of the League for the Hard of Hearing. These headphones can be used when the plane has a jack to accommodate the headphone plug. Older planes do not all have such jacks, but new planes usually do. Available at Sam Ash and other audio stores; cost: $90

Listening Systems: Group and Others

FM INTERCOM: DeVilbiss Development Co., Ltd., 3056 Hazelton St., Falls Church, VA 22044; phone: 703-534-1681; cost: approximately $75

AREA LOOPS: Oval Window Audio, 33 Wildflower Court, Nederland, CO 80466; phone (voice or text telephone): 303-447-3607; cost: approximately $700

MANUAL ALPHABET

Telephone Aids

AMPLIFICATION WHEEL VOLUME CONTROL HANDSET: AT&T Special Needs Center; phone: 800-233-1222; cost: approximately $35. The AT&T Volume Control Handset costs $35. The entire phone with Handset that does not have volume control costs $40 for the rotary dial, $50 for touch-tone. People with hearing impairment would replace the regular handset with the Volume Control Handset. The total cost is $75 or $85.

PORTABLE AMPLIFIER: AT&T Special Needs Center or Radio Shack; cost: approximately $11

CLARITY PHONE: Walker Equipment, Highway 151 South, Ringgold, GA 30736; phone: 800-426-3738; cost: approximately $150; can also be purchased through audiologists

COMTEK TELEPHONE ADAPTER: Comtek, 357 West 2700 South, Salt Lake City, UT 84115 (includes Comtek companion listening system); cost: approximately $800

TEXT TELEPHONE (TTY; also called TELECOMMUNICATION DEVICE FOR THE DEAF or TDD; phone messages are typed): TTY Inc., 202 Lexington Ave., Hackensack, NJ 07601; cost: $189–$600
AT&T Special Needs Center; cost: $200–$400

Ultratec, 450 Science Dr, Madison, WI 53711; phone: 608-238-5400; cost: $299 plus shipping ($7).

TELELINK (used with Pocketalker): Williams Sound Corporation; phone: 800-328-6190; cost: approximately $40

TELETALKER TELEPHONE: Williams Sound Corporation; cost: audiologist fitted, $399; not fitted, $299

Financial Community Assists to People with Hearing Impairment

A Merrill Lynch national program, run by Christopher Sullivan and his associate, Kelly Les, trains financial executives to help people with hearing handicaps. Financial executives are trained in the special uses of the telephone and other assistive devices, including text telephones; phone: 609-282-1673; text telephone: 609-282-1944.

Television Aids

INFRARED SYSTEM: Sound Associates, 424 W. 45 St., NY 10036; cost: approximately $300

TELECAPTION DECODER: Units (16" by 8" by 4") are available at Service Merchandise, through the Sears and Penney's catalogues, and at more than a thousand retail outlets. For rebates and other information, contact the National Captioning Institute; toll-free numbers: voice phone (800-533-9673) and TTY phone (800-321-8337); cost: approximately $200

Safety Aids

SILENT CALL (lights lamps, vibrates; for phone, door, fire alarm, baby): Silent Call, Clarkston, MI; phone: 313-391-1710; cost: $350–$600

SILENT PAGE WRIST ALERT (vibrates as an alert for any area of the home): Sawtech Communications, Inc. *(Sawtech has most assistive devices.);* voice phone: 718-793-6929; TTY: 718-454-6911; cost: approximately $350

SMOKE ALARM REPEATER (light goes on and off): TTY INC.; phone: 201-489-7889; cost: $35–$38

SONY STEREO HEADPHONE sometimes picks up announcements by airline pilot

DELUXE VIBRATING ALARM CLOCK: Hal-Hen Co.; phone: 800-221-0188; cost: $130

SUPER DRI-AID (removes damaging moisture from in-the-ear hearing aids): Hal-Hen Co.; phone: 800-221-0188; cost: $14.95

Nonlisting of other assistive devices in no way impugns the excellence of other assistive devices. Read *Silent News* and *SHHH* journals or contact *Gallaudet Assistive Devices Center* (Gallaudet University) for information about the latest equipment. Or contact Sound Waves, a new company that sells most assistive devices, at P.O. Box 563, New Rochelle, NY 10802; phone: 914-632-8140 voice and TTY.

Organizations

a.b.c. Advocates for Better Communication*
71 W. 23 St.
New York, NY 10010

* Advocates for Better Communication/a.b.c. is a volunteer group allied with the League for the Hard of Hearing, whose mission,

Alexander Graham Bell Association for the Deaf
3417 Volta Place NW
Washington, DC 20007

American Speech-Language-Hearing Association
10801 Rockville Pike
Rockville, MD 20852

American Tinnitus Association
P.O. Box 5
Portland, OR 97207

American Academy of Otolaryngology
  Head and Neck Surgery
1101 Vermont Ave. NW, Suite 302
Washington, DC 20005

Better Hearing Institute
5021B Backlick Rd.
Annandale, VA 22003

The Deafness Research Foundation
9 East 38th Street
New York, NY 10016

Gallaudet University
800 Florida Ave. NE
Washington, DC 20002

Hard of Hearing Advocates (hard of hearing awareness
  kits for hospitals and medical facilities)
245 Prospect Street
Framingham, MA 01701

---

through education and advocacy, is to make it possible for people
with all degrees of hearing loss to participate fully in society.

National Hearing Aid Society
20361 Middlebelt Rd.
Livonia, MI 48152

National Captioning Institute
5203 Leesburg Pike, Suite 1500
Falls Church, VA 22041

National Institute on Deafness and Other
  Communication Disorders
P.O. Box 37777
Washington, DC 20013-7777

League for the Hard of Hearing
71 West 23 St.
New York, NY 10010-4162

Self Help for Hard of Hearing People, Inc. (SHHH)
7910 Woodmont Ave.
Bethesda, MD 20814

Facilities Providing Total Service for the Hard-of-Hearing

- The House Ear Clinic, Inc., 256 South Lake Street, Los Angeles, CA 90057.
- Kresge Hearing Research Laboratory of the South, Louisiana State University Medical Center, 2020 Gravier Street, New Orleans, LA 70112-2234.
- Kresge Hearing Research Institute, University of Michigan Medical Center, 1904 Taubman Health Care Center, Ann Arbor, Michigan, 48109-0312.
- League for the Hard of Hearing, 71 West 23 Street, New York, NY 10010.
- Oregon Hearing Research Center, Oregon Health

Sciences University, 3515 S.W. Veterans Hospital Road, Portland, Oregon 97201-2997.

Publications for the Hearing-Impaired

Silent News, P.O. Box 23330, Rochester, NY 14692-3330 (yearly subscription, $15)

The SHHH Journal, available from Self Help for Hard of Hearing People, Inc., 7800 Wisconsin Ave., Bethesda, MD 20814 (yearly subscription and membership dues, $20)

Communication Assistive Devices, a booklet from the House Ear Institute, 256 South Lake St., Los Angeles, CA 90057 (no charge).

a.b.c. REPORTS, a publication of Advocates for Better Communication, 71 West 29 St., New York, NY 10010-4162

Relay Customer Services Directory
(Compiled by TDI)

The following are customer service numbers for relay services. Call those numbers if you have questions, complaints, problems, or even to say thank you.
Please inform TDI of any additions, deletions, or corrections.

Statewide			
Alabama	*205-987-4410	Louisiana	*800-333-0605	Puerto Rico	800-682-8786
Alaska	*907-376-6770	Maine	703-679-5977	Rhode Island	800-659-2905
Arizona	800-347-1695	Maryland	800-377-1120	South Carolina	800-377-1170
Arkansas	800-285-7192	Massachusetts	*508-460-3910	South Dakota	800-377-1180
California	800-377-1140	Michigan	800-432-5413	Tennessee	*615-371-5624
	*916-928-3400	Minnesota	*612-297-6711	Texas	800-578-6275
Colorado	800-377-1130	Mississippi	*800-557-7755	Utah	801-262-3931
Connecticut	800-659-2905	Missouri	800-377-1180	Vermont	703-679-5977
		Montana	703-679-5977	Virgin Islands	800-682-8786
		Nebraska	*800-322-5299	Virginia	703-679-5977

Delaware	703-679-5977	Nevada	800-377-1130	Washington	*206-441-2000

State	Number	State	Number	State	Number
Delaware	703-679-5977	Nevada	800-377-1130	Washington	*206-441-2000
District of Columbia	202-434-1781	New Hampshire	800-377-1160	West Virginia	*518-383-7018
Florida	*800-955-8013	New Jersey	609-581-3925	Wisconsin	800-283-9877
Georgia	*404-729-5005	New Mexico	800-377-1130	Wyoming	800-377-1180
Hawaii	*808-945-3533	New York	*518-383-7018		
Idaho	*800-368-6185	North Carolina	800-377-1170	**Nationwide Long Distance Customer Services**	
Illinois	703-679-5977	North Dakota	800-377-1180		
Indiana	800-377-1101	Ohio	216-476-6002	AT&T	800-682-8786
Iowa	800-377-1190	Oklahoma	800-217-3848	MCI	800-374-4833
Kansas	*913-865-3271	Oregon	800-377-1150	Sprint	*800-676-3777
Kentucky	*205-987-4410	Pennsylvania	215-975-3621		

* = Voice & TTY B = Telebraille C = Computer V = Voice Only Blank = TTY LD = Long Distance

Telecommunications Relay Services Directory

(Compiled by TDI)

The following are relay services that are available 24 hours a day, 7 days a week, and 365 days a year. Please inform TDI of any additions, deletions, or corrections.

Statewide			
Alabama	800-548-2546 800-548-2547/V	Louisiana	800-846-5277 800-947-5277/V
Alaska	800-770-8973 800-770-8255/V	Maine	800-437-1220 800-457-1220/V
Arizona	800-367-8939 800-842-4681/V	Maryland	*800-735-2258
Arkansas	800-285-1131 800-285-1121/V	Massachusetts	*800-439-2370
California	800-735-2929 800-735-2922/V	Michigan	*800-649-3777
Colorado	800-659-2656 800-659-3656/V 800-659-4656/C	Minnesota Mpls-St.Paul	*800-627-3529 612-297-5353
Connecticut	800-842-9710 800-833-8134/V	Mississippi	*800-582-2233
		Missouri	800-735-2966 800-735-2466/V
		Montana	800-253-4091 800-253-4093/V
		Nebraska	800-833-7352 800-833-0920/V

Rhode Island	*800-745-5555		
South Carolina	*800-735-2905		
South Dakota	*800-877-1113		
Tennessee	800-848-0298 800-848-0299/V		
Texas	800-735-2989 800-735-2988/V 800-735-2991/C		
Utah	*800-346-4128		
Salt Lake	*801-298-9484		
Ogden	*801-546-2982		
Logan	*801-752-9596		
Provo-Orem	*801-374-2504		
Vermont	800-253-0191 800-253-0195/V		
Virgin Islands	800-440-8477 800-809-8477/V		

State	Numbers		State	Numbers
Delaware	800-232-5460 800-232-5470/V		Nevada	800-326-6868 800-326-6888/V
District of Columbia	202-855-1234 202-855-1000/V		New Hampshire	*800-735-2964
Florida	800-955-8771 800-955-8770/V		New Jersey	800-852-7899 800-852-7897/V
Georgia	800-255-0056 800-255-0135/V		New Mexico	800-659-8331 800-659-1779/V
Hawaii	711 511/V 808-643-8833 808-546-2565/V		New York	800-662-1220 800-421-1220/V
Idaho	800-377-3529 800-377-1363/V		North Carolina	800-735-2962 800-735-8262/V
Illinois	800-526-0844 800-526-0857/V		North Dakota	800-366-6888 800-366-6889/V
Indiana	*800-743-3333		Ohio	*800-750-0750
Iowa	800-735-2942 800-735-2943/V		Oklahoma	*800-722-0353/N *800-522-8506/S
Kansas	*800-766-3777		Oregon	*800-735-2900
Kentucky	800-648-6056 800-648-6057/V		Pennsylvania	800-654-5984 800-654-5988/V
			Puerto Rico	800-240-2050 800-260-2050/V 800-208-2828/LD 800-290-2828/V/LD

State	Numbers
Virginia	800-828-1120 800-828-1140/V
Washington	800-833-6388 800-833-6384/V 800-833-6385/B
West Virginia	800-982-8771 800-982-8772/V
Wisconsin	*800-947-3529
Wyoming	800-877-9965 800-877-9975/V

Nationwide Long Distance Relay Services

Service	Numbers
AT&T	800-855-2880 800-855-2881/V 800-855-2882/C 800-855-2883/B
Hamilton	*800-833-5833
MCI	800-688-4889 800-947-8642/V
Sprint	*800-877-8973

* = Voice & TTY   B = Telebraille   C = Computer   V = Voice Only   Blank = TTY   LD = Long Distance

Author's Afterword

The Overview of the Americans with Disabilities Act (ADA) of 1989 was passed by the Senate September 7, 1989.

"The purpose of the ADA is to provide a clear and comprehensive national mandate to end discrimination against individuals with disabilities, and to ensure that the Federal government plays a central role in enforcing these standards on behalf of individuals with disabilities."*

In July 1990 The Americans With Disabilities Act (ADA) was signed into law.

This gift was given to people with hearing impairment five years after I began interviewing and doing research for *When the Hearing Gets Hard*. In revising and updating this book for paperback, I have enumerated the benefits of the ADA to the millions with hearing disorders.

Now the ultimate gift to people with certain hearing disorders—the gift of regenerated sensory cells so that sensorineural "nerve" impairment becomes reversible—

* Bob Silverstein, Staff Director & Chief counsel, Subcommittee on Disability Policy, Senator Tom Harkin, Chair

is being hinted at. It is my hope that five years hence, when I update *When the Hearing Gets Hard* once again, the gift of regenerated sensory cells will be a reality, a gift to be celebrated as we now celebrate the Americans with Disabilities Act.

References

Brummett, R. E. *Review Article Otolaryngologic Side Effects of Drugs.* Portland, OR: Skyline /pharmIndex, August 1991.

Davies, D. M. *FRCP Textbook of Adverse Drug Reactions.* 3rd ed. New York: Oxford University Press, 1985.

Drug Interactions and Side Effects Index (keyed to *Physicians' Desk Reference).* Montvale, NJ: Medical Economics, 1991.

Dukes, M. N. G., ed. *Meyler's Side Effects of Drugs: An Encyclopedia of Adverse Reactions and Interactions.* Amsterdam: Elsevier, 1988.

English, G. M. *Otolaryngology.* rev. ed. Philadelphia: Harper & Row, 1983.

Harpur E. S. *Disorders of the Ear: Iatrogenic Diseases.* 3rd ed. Oxford: Oxford Press, 1986.

Hawkins, J. E., V. Beger, J. Aran. *"Antibiotic Insults to Corti's Organ."* In *Sensorineural Hearing Processes and Disorders,* edited by A. B. Graham. Boston: Little, Brown, 1967.

Hawkins, J. E. *Drug Ototoxicity: Handbook of Sensory Physiology.* Vol. 5, Part 3. Berlin: Springer Verlag, 1976.

Hawkins, J. E., L. G. Johnsson, W. C. Stebbins, D. B. Moody, and S. L. Coombs. "Hearing Loss and Cochlear

Pathology in Monkeys After Noise Exposure." *Acta Oto-Laryngologica* 81(1976): 337–343.

Hawkins, J. E., L. Johnsson. "Otopathological Changes Associated with Presbyacusia." *Seminars in Hearing* 6 (1985): 115–133.

Hawkins, J. E., A. G. D. Maran, and P. M. Stell, eds. "Ototoxicity." Chap. 7 in *Clinical Otolaryngology*. Cambridge, MA: Blackwell Scientific, 1979.

Hawkins, J. E. *Ototoxicity in Infant and Fetus: Childhood Deafness*. Philadelphia: Grune & Stratton, 1977.

Hotchkiss, D. *Demographic Aspects of Hearing Impairment: Questions and Answers*. 2nd ed. Washington, DC: Center for Assessment and Demographic Studies, Gallaudet Research Institute, 1989.

Jinks, M. J. *Counseling Older Adults with Hearing Impairment*. Port Washington, NY: Pharmacy Times, 1990.

Lee, K. J., ed. *Essential Otolaryngology: Head and Neck Surgery*. 3rd ed. New Hyde Park, NY: Medical Examination, 1983.

Lerner, S. A., G. J. Matz, and J. E. Hawkins. *Aminoglycoside Ototoxicity*. Boston: Little, Brown, 1977.

Miller, J. J. *Handbook of Ototoxicity*. Boca Raton, FL: CRC Press, 1985.

National Institute on Deafness and Other Communication Disorders. *National Strategic Research Plan*. Bethesda, MD: National Institutes of Health, 1989.

National Institutes of Health. *Hearing Loss* (NIH Publication No 82-157). Bethesda, MD: U.S. Department of Health and Human Services, January 1982.

Norris, C. H. *Drugs 36: Drugs Affecting the Inner Ear: A Review of Their Clinical Efficacy*. Langhorne, PA: Adis Press Limited, 1988.

Physicians' Desk Reference. 45th ed. Montvale, NJ: Medical Economics, 1991.

Stringer, S. P., W. L. Meyerhoff, and C. G. Wright. "Diseases of the Ear." In *Otolaryngology* (Vol. 2), edited by Paparella, Chap. 46. Philadelphia: W. B. Saunders, 1991.

Van Cleve, John V., ed. *Gallaudet Encyclopedia of Deaf People and Deafness.* New York: McGraw-Hill, 1987.

Walker, E. M., M. A. Fazekas-May, and W. R. Bowen. *Nephrotoxic and Ototoxic Agents (Clinical Toxicology I): Clinics in Laboratory Medicine (Vol. 10, No. 2).* Little Rock, AR: John L. McClellan Memorial VA Hospital, June 1990.

Index

About the Author

Elaine Suss, a novelist, poet, and journalist, was motivated to write this book by her recent severe hearing loss. In addition to *When the Hearing Gets Hard*, she has published articles on auditory loss, and poetry, in *Newsday*, *Saturday Review*, *The Cleveland Plain Dealer*, *Christian Science Monitor*, and many literary magazines. She is also the author of the novel *A Money Marriage*. In an appearance on CBS *This Morning*, she exposed the deafening effects of many common medications. Ms. Suss and her husband reside in Great Neck, New York, and in New York City. They have two children and five grandchildren.